Women and Cardiovascular Disease

Addressing Disparities in Care

Women and Cardiovascular Disease

Addressing Disparities in Care

Kevin R Campbell, MD, FACC

University of North Carolina, USA

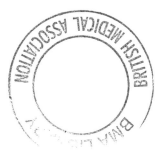

Imperial College Press

Published by

Imperial College Press
57 Shelton Street
Covent Garden
London WC2H 9HE

Distributed by

World Scientific Publishing Co. Pte. Ltd.
5 Toh Tuck Link, Singapore 596224
USA office: 27 Warren Street, Suite 401-402, Hackensack, NJ 07601
UK office: 57 Shelton Street, Covent Garden, London WC2H 9HE

Library of Congress Cataloging-in-Publication Data
Campbell, Kevin R., author.
    Women and cardiovascular disease : addressing disparities in care / Kevin R. Campbell.
        p. ; cm.
    Includes bibliographical references and index.
    ISBN 978-1-78326-500-8 (hardcover : alk. paper) -- ISBN 978-1-78326-501-5 (pbk. : alk. paper)
    I. Title.
    [DNLM: 1. Cardiovascular Diseases--therapy. 2. Women. 3. Healthcare Disparities. 4. Sex
Factors. 5. Treatment Outcome. WG 166]
    RA645.C34
    616.10082--dc23
                                                            2014034450

British Library Cataloguing-in-Publication Data
A catalogue record for this book is available from the British Library.

Typeset by Stallion Press
Email: enquiries@stallionpress.com

Printed in Singapore

Dedication

This book is dedicated to the women in my life. My wife and daughter inspire me on a daily basis. They have endured countless days of writing and revising manuscripts and have supported me throughout my journey to completion. It is my hope that this book will educate and engage others and ultimately improve cardiovascular care for women all over the world.

My daughter, Bek, designed and created the cover art for this book. As one of millions of people throughout the world with type 1 insulin-dependent diabetes, she battles chronic disease on a daily basis and handles all of the challenges diabetes brings with a maturity beyond her years as well as a quiet grace. This book is my gift to Bek — when I am no longer here to advocate for her, it is my hope that there will be healthcare professionals that are armed with the information they need to aggressively treat and prevent needless cardiovascular deaths and disease in women. Moreover, I hope that this book will serve to engage and motivate other women to take control of their own heart health.

About the Artist

Bek Campbell is a middle-school student in Raleigh, NC. She enjoys the visual and performing arts, including drawing, digital art, photography, singing in the school show choir and playing guitar. While leaving her career choices open at this point, Bek has a strong interest in film making.

Bek also enjoys animals and volunteers at a local animal shelter assisting the shelter veterinarian with prepping and caring for cats undergoing surgical procedures. Bek is the proud parent of four rescue animals: three cats and a dog.

About the Author

Dr Kevin R Campbell, MD, FACC is an assistant professor of medicine at the University of North Carolina at Chapel Hill in the division of cardiovascular medicine. Dr Campbell received his undergraduate degree in biochemistry from North Carolina State University and his medical degree from Wake Forest University. He then completed his residency training in internal medicine at the University of Virginia and fellowships in cardiology and cardiac electrophysiology at Duke University.

Dr Campbell is an internationally recognized expert in the prevention of sudden cardiac death in women. Inspired by his wife and daughter, Dr Campbell is passionate about addressing gender disparities in cardiovascular care and speaks to healthcare providers all over the US in order to raise awareness for the treatment of heart disease in women.

In addition to his clinical activities, Dr Campbell is an on-air media expert and is the in-studio medical expert for WNCN TV in Raleigh, NC. He also is an on-air contributor for Fox News Channel and the Fox Business Channel, and appears live on national television to provide insight into breaking medical stories as well as commentary on healthcare policy.

Contents

Introduction

Cardiovascular disease is the number one killer of both men and women in the US and in the UK today. Many of us are unaware of the risk factors and potential impacts of this potentially fatal disease and most are unprepared when it strikes. Due to advances in medical science and technology over the last 20 years, cardiovascular disease is now a very treatable condition and cardiovascular death is often preventable. Nonetheless, it remains a serious public health problem of epidemic proportions. It is imperative that both caregivers and patients understand the various ways in which cardiovascular disease may present and progress throughout the disease process — particularly when it comes to differences based on gender. In order to illustrate this broad range of clinical presentations, I believe it is important that we begin our discussion, and this book, with two very dichotomous cases.

Bob is a 50-year-old man with a family of three. He owns a small office supply business in town. A long-time fixture in the community, he provides office supplies and equipment to companies all over the city. He has many long-standing customers and provides personalized services such as delivery and set up. Over the last several years, it has become increasingly difficult to compete with the big "chain" office supply stores. The larger corporate stores are able to undercut his pricing and he has begun to lose customers. He watches his profit margins fall and his expenses rise. His work hours increase as he is forced to lay off several employees. He no longer exercises and begins to smoke more heavily. Over the last six months he has gained nearly 25 pounds. He is no longer able to afford health insurance and has not seen a physician in over two years. This morning, he rushes into the office to meet with suppliers who no longer want to provide his store with inventory. As he sits at his desk, he begins to sweat. He is breathing heavily and begins to feel a tightness in his chest. The pain in his chest intensifies and then he slumps face first onto his desk. The staff quickly calls 911 and begins an attempt at CPR. Bob is transported to the local emergency room and is found by the emergency medical system (EMS) first responders to be in ventricular fibrillation with evidence of ST elevation in the anterior leads. Luckily he is revived with defibrillation en route. On arrival at the hospital, the cardiologist is alerted and the cardiac catheterization laboratory is prepared for urgent primary percutaneous coronary intervention (PCI). Bob arrives in the catheterization laboratory and is found to have a 99% lesion in his left anterior descending (LAD) artery and undergoes primary stenting with an excellent result. A few days later, he is fully recovered with normal left ventricular function and is released from the hospital with a good medical regimen and a plan for secondary prevention.

Cindy is a 47-year-old mother of three and wife to a banking executive. Formally, Cindy worked as an attorney but retired in order to be a full-time mother to her children. She is active in the community and volunteers at her childrens' schools and also enjoys gardening in her yard. She exercises regularly and is in relatively good shape. She has had "borderline" high blood pressure for several years but her physician has not yet initiated drug therapy. Her dad died suddenly in his 50s but no one ever knew why or what happened. Lately she has been feeling a bit fatigued but she has attributed it to her busy schedule with the kids. In addition, Cindy has noticed a feeling of "dread" from time to time over the last few weeks. Sometimes she feels as though something is just "not right" and easily becomes anxious. Sometimes when she is exercising, she notices a heaviness in her chest that seems to get better when she takes a deep breath and rests for a bit. She notices a similar sensation in her chest when she is rushing around in the morning trying to help her three kids get ready for school. Her symptoms continue to occur and begin to increase in frequency. She begins to think that she is just "run-down" from her busy schedule and makes an appointment to see her gynecologist (who she uses as a primary care doctor) because she thinks she may have the flu. After three days, she is able to see her doctor. Her doctor quickly prescribes her an antidepressant as well as an anxiolytic and postulates that she maybe nearing an early menopause and experiencing symptoms of a mid-life crisis. He tells her that her chest heaviness may be related to panic attacks or hormonal imbalances. He draws blood tests to evaluate her for evidence of menopause and schedules an appointment in six weeks to assess the effects of the antidepressants. That night, Cindy is cooking dinner when she suddenly falls to the floor. EMS is alerted and when they arrive, she is pulseless and they are unable to revive her. Due to the unexplained death, an autopsy is performed where Cindy is found to have a 75% left-main lesion with what appears to be a freshly ruptured plaque. Cause of death was determined to be a massive myocardial infarction.

Two scenarios with two very different outcomes — one happy ending and one very unfortunate result leaving three children without a mother. Why? How could Cindy's outcome have been impacted and her life spared?

Traditionally, cardiovascular disease and sudden cardiac death has been thought of as a disease of men. Public perception of the classic cardiac patient in the US today is that of a middle-aged, overweight male who smokes and works long hours in a stressful job. This image is supported by the way in which media portrays the victims of cardiovascular disease to the public. For instance, when watching medical dramas on television the character that is most often rushed to the emergency room with classic symptoms of chest pain only to arrest and die after heroic resuscitative efforts by the ER staff is almost always male — leaving behind a grieving wife and child. However, both men and women are at risk for cardiovascular disease and its related complications. Although our biology is different hormonally, much of the way in which coronary artery disease develops is similar in both sexes.

The fact is that more women than men die each year from cardiovascular disease. Data from the American Heart Association has shown that mortality rates for men with heart disease have improved where those of women have either declined or remained the same. The same statistics are seen in the UK as well as in the other industrialized nations in Europe. Advocacy and educational efforts continue to lag far behind the ever-expanding gender gap in cardiac care. Government agencies and policy makers in both government and industry are not doing enough to help close the gap. Former First Lady Laura Bush addressed the American College of Cardiology in 2004 and got it right when she stated, "with the many risk factors for cardiovascular disease, a woman's greatest risk is ignorance".[1]

The undeniable truth is that women are undertreated and underserved with respect to prevention, diagnosis and treatment of cardiovascular disease. Women's symptoms are often minimized and attributed to stress, anxiety or other psychiatric diseases. In order to impact this disparity in care and effect change we must educate and improve awareness amongst physicians, physician extenders and other caregivers. We must improve awareness of risk for cardiovascular disease in women (and their families and loved ones) all over the world.

Why is this? Who is responsible? How can we as healthcare providers and healthcare consumers impact this chasm in care?

Over the last 20 years, much has been done to improve survival rates from cardiovascular disease. Technological advances have

---

[1]Former First Lady Laura Bush's Plenary Address to the American College of Cardiology Meetings in New Orleans, March 2004.

provided physicians and healthcare workers with tools that can significantly reduce morbidity and mortality. Now, when a patient presents with an acute coronary syndrome (ACS), the cardiac catheterization laboratory can be activated and the patient can undergo percutaneous revascularization (primary stenting) within 45 minutes from the time of presentation. Data supports the improved outcomes and myocardial salvage in ACS when prompt revascularization occurs. However, as you will come to discover through the course of this book, data over the last ten years demonstrate a gender gap. Men tend to be treated with more aggressive tools and procedures when presenting with a similar clinical scenario as compared to women. In addition, preventative efforts have expanded to address risk factors such as hyperlipidemia, hypertension, tobacco abuse and sedentary lifestyle much earlier. However, these preventative efforts are not always applied to both men and women with similar urgency and aggressiveness.

There are many advocacy efforts underway in the US today such as the American Heart Association's "Go Red for Women" campaign — but this is not enough. The majority of women still do not realize that their greatest risk of death is coronary artery disease. Most women still believe that they will ultimately succumb to breast or uterine cancer instead. More importantly, the medical community as a whole does not do enough to narrow the gender gap we see in cardiovascular care.

As healthcare professionals, we all learn best when we approach problems in a case-based fashion. Much research in medical education over the last 20 years has shown that we learn better and retain more information for practical use when we learn it in association with a clinical scenario or patient interaction. In fact, many medical schools in the US today have moved to a blended case-based curriculum rather than a lecture hall format. As clinicians, we are all trained to focus on the patient and on the clinical signs and symptoms that have led that particular person to seek evaluation. In each chapter I will present real-world cases in order to illustrate points of emphasis and relate our discussion to the reason we all practice (or hope to practice) medicine — the patient.

During the course of the book, we will explore the scope of the problem and attempt to understand why disparities exist. We will discuss the biological differences in coronary artery disease in men and women, how presentations vary and how specific types of testing and diagnostic evaluations are more or less accurate in men versus women. We will discuss the impact that OB-GYN physicians can have on improving women's cardiovascular health. Although traditionally, OB-GYN physicians have focused on reproductive health, these practitioners may, in fact, be the key to narrowing the gap in care. As we go through the issues associated with the gender disparities in cardiac care, we will postulate as to the root causes and offer potential solutions. Most importantly, we will discuss ways in which we can empower women to impact their own cardiovascular health throughout their lives.

This book is intended to make a difference. This book is personal. This book is for my daughter Bek. At age five, Bek developed insulin-dependent diabetes. Unless a cure for diabetes is provided in her lifetime, she will certainly experience the ravages of cardiovascular disease one day. I want to make it my business to ensure that there are well-educated, non-biased medical professionals to care for her in a non-gender-biased way when she develops symptoms or disease. The goal of this book is to be a first step in narrowing the gender gap in cardiovascular care. Ultimately, this book is designed to open the eyes of healthcare providers — medical professionals and practitioners and policy makers — it should serve as a "call to action" to promote better cardiovascular care for all individuals, irrespective of gender.

Chapter One

Epidemiologic Considerations in Cardiovascular Disease

Cardiovascular disease is the number one killer of both men and women in the industrialized world today. Even if we combine all deaths from all types of cancers and HIV-related illness there are more deaths from heart disease. No longer a disease exclusive to men, just over half of all cardiac-related deaths are in women. In the last year, nearly 8.5 million women worldwide died of heart disease and this accounted for one third of all female deaths. Heart disease and heart-disease-related deaths are epidemic: one person dies of heart disease every 33 seconds in the US today.

Obviously, heart disease and its complications remain a major international public health problem. Although great progress has been made over the last 20 years, too many people are dying. Medicine has made great strides in diagnosis, prevention and treatment of cardiovascular disease. However, as healthcare providers, we are not doing enough. Efforts at prevention before disease and risk factor modification after disease presentation are not going far enough — patients are still not being screened and risk factors are not being modified. We must do more to prevent disease and identify those at risk, whether male or female. Awareness and advocacy efforts are lacking and patients are going untreated. In fact, most women consider their greatest risk of death to be from cancers of the breast, ovaries or uterus — in actuality, cardiovascular disease is the number one killer of women worldwide.

According to the Centers for Disease Control (CDC), there are approximately 800,000 deaths annually from cardiovascular disease in the US. Of these, nearly 210,000 deaths are preventable. In the UK and throughout Europe, the percentage of cardiovascular deaths are quite similar. The *European Heart Journal* reported this year that heart disease is the leading cause of death in Europe and accounts for 46% of all fatalities and affects over 4 million individuals.[1] Women represent a significant proportion of cardiac-related death and a substantial number of them are, in fact, preventable. Data from the American Heart Association indicates that 1 in 3 females are living with heart disease today. Since 1984, deaths in women have exceeded those of males.[2] Interestingly, during this same time period, only 25–30% of all patients treated with either percutaneous coronary intervention (PCI) or coronary artery bypass grafting (CABG) were female. Nearly 6.6 million women are living with heart disease in the US today and almost two thirds of those who die suddenly have no prior symptoms of disease. Most women do not even know that they are at risk. In Europe, the numbers of deaths in women attributable to heart disease exceeds those of men — in fact, 51% of females deaths are from cardiovascular disease and only 42% of deaths in men are from cardiovascular disease. As expected, the rates of heart disease and cardiovascular death do vary from country to country in Europe. As a whole, death rates are declining throughout the world but obviously substantial morbidity and mortality still exists.

[1] Nichols, M., Townsend, N., Scarborough, P. *et al.* (2013). European Cardiovascular Disease Statistics 4th edition 2012: EuroHeart II, *Eur Heart J*, Volume 34, 3007–3013.

[2] Go, A. S., Mozaffarian, D., Roger, V. L. *et al.* (2013). Heart disease and stroke statistics — 2013 update: A report from the American Heart Association. *Circulation*, Volume 127, e6–e245.

Recently, a report was released in the US that detailed the fact that preventable deaths from heart disease have declined in older persons but have not declined at nearly the same rate in younger populations (particularly those under the age of 65).[3] This is particularly concerning in that it provides clear evidence that we are not doing enough work in prevention in younger patient populations. The fact that preventable deaths are not declining in the younger cohort suggests that physicians and other healthcare providers must do a better job of aggressively screening for and treating of risk factors in patients at earlier ages — even in the 20s and 30s. In this report, rates of preventable cardiovascular deaths declined by 29% in those 75 and younger — however, when the younger population was examined (particularly those in the 40–65 age group) it was found that only 48% of those with high cholesterol were actually treated. Moreover, nearly 29% of these patients were smokers as compared to only 5% in the over-65 category. Older persons tend to have more opportunities for interaction with physicians due to the fact that they often have a larger number of accumulated medical problems requiring regular follow-up care. In contrast, younger adults feel invincible and give almost no thought to prevention or their own mortality. The data is clear — we must change the attitudes of both physicians and patients in order to make an impact in preventable death rates.

In women, these numbers are even more staggering. Although biologically different with a discordant hormonal milieu from men, women present a large number of cases of cardiovascular disease and sudden cardiac death. As previously mentioned, heart disease may present differently in women and may be more difficult to detect and recognize. Women are less likely to seek treatment as compared to men. Women who do seek care are much often treated less aggressively often due to atypical presentations and

---

[3] Centers for Disease Control and Prevention (2013). Vital signs: avoidable deaths from heart disease, stroke, and hypertensive disease — US, 2001–2010. *MMWR*, Volume 62(35), 721–727.

predetermined attitudes about women presenting with cardiac-like symptoms.

Cardiovascular disease encompasses all of the diseases of the blood vessels heart and lungs. The leading cause of death from cardiovascular disease is coronary artery disease. Coronary artery disease (CAD) is the number one killer of men and women in the US today. Major risk factors for CAD include diabetes, hypertension, hyperlipidemia, tobacco abuse and positive family history for CAD. Other risk factors include metabolic syndrome, obesity and sedentary lifestyle. There have been multiple public campaigns in the US and throughout the UK aimed at raising awareness of risk factors and motivating potential patients to effect lifestyle changes.

This year in *Circulation*, an update on 2013 rates of cardiovascular disease and stroke was published by the American Heart Association (AHA) and the results were quite surprising.[2] In spite of efforts to increase awareness, rates of high-risk behaviors continue. With the innovations in diagnosis and treatment available to patients and physicians in the US and in the UK there should be no reason for increasing rates of risk factor prevalence. However, that is not the case.

Smoking

For example, over 20% of men and nearly 17% of women continue to smoke in the US today. According to the British Heart Foundation, 20% of adults continue to smoke. Smoking results in inflammation and damage to the endothelial lining of blood vessels including the coronary arteries and plays a key role in the development of atherosclerotic plaques. On a positive note, the rates of exposure to second-hand smoke of non-smokers has fallen nearly 10% over the same time period — likely due to the passage of smoking bans in public places in many states throughout the US. Other risk factors continue to be ignored as well.

Cholesterol/Hyperlipidemia

According to the CDC the number of adults in the US with cholesterol levels above 240 mg/dL remains at nearly 32 million individuals. In the UK, more than 60% of men and more than 65% of women have high cholesterol. Most are not adequately treated. Chronically elevated serum cholesterol levels leads to deposition in the coronary arteries and development of plaques that may eventually rupture and result in an acute myocardial infarction (AMI). Diet and lifestyle play a critical role in the development of hyperlipidemia and genetic factors predispose patients to higher cholesterol levels requiring drug therapy.

Hypertension

Today, the incidence of hypertension approaches 35%. Of those with hypertension about 75% are aware of their condition but only 50% have their blood pressure under adequate control. Hypertension appears to affect both men and women equally but more men than women are on therapy at any one time. Hypertension results in the loss of compliance of arteries and can result in stiffness and further endothelial damage and inflammation. Untreated or undertreated hypertension can result in damage to other organs including the brain, kidneys, eyes as well as the heart and circulatory system. Those of lower socioeconomic status and those from certain ethnic groups such as Hispanics and African Americans tend to be treated at a lower rate and have a higher incidence of disease. Estimates from the British Heart Foundation indicate that nearly 5 million people are living in the UK with undiagnosed and untreated hypertension — which puts them at significant risk for heart disease.

Diabetes

Diabetes is seen in nearly 9% of the US population (19 million Americans) and another 8 million people have undiagnosed diabetes with almost 30% of people having the syndrome of "pre-diabetes" with high fasting blood glucose levels and evidence of insulin resistance. It is concerning that the incidence of diabetes is increasing significantly in the US today. The largest increase is in type 2 (adult onset diabetes) and appears to be directly related to the epidemic rate of obesity in the US and Europe today. The metabolic affects of long-standing, poorly controlled diabetes significantly contributes to the development of atherosclerotic plaques in the coronary arteries.

Obesity

Obesity in both the US and in the UK continues to pose a major public health problem. Last year, obesity-related illness accounted for nearly 150 billion dollars of healthcare spending in the US alone. Obesity contributes to the development of diabetes, hypertension and high cholesterol. According to the University of Birmingham in the UK, nearly 25% of the British population are considered obese and the numbers continue to rise.[4] A Gallup poll conducted in the US in 2013 has shown a steady increase in obesity rates with nearly 27% of Americans now considered obese (as defined by a BMI over 30) and more than 35% are considered overweight.

The rate of rise in obesity appears to be similar in both men and women and across all demographic groups. It appears that we are a culture of over-indulgence and, through poor habits, continue to put ourselves at increased risk for heart disease.

Fortunately, overall death rates in the US from heart disease (across all groups) are declining — however, the burden of disease and the prevalence of risk factors attributable to disease continue to rise. Each year nearly 400,000 Americans die from heart disease and nearly 700,000 Americans experience a heart attack — another 150,000 have a silent, asymptomatic coronary event. One in six

---

[4] Reported on the University of Birmingham website. http://www.birmingham.ac.uk/research/activity/mds/centres/obesity/obesity-uk/index.aspx. Accessed 15 April 2014.

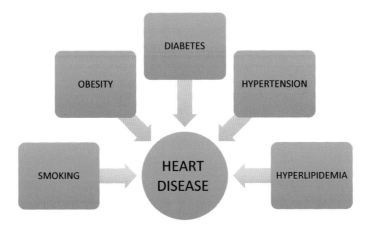

Figure 1.1 High-risk behaviors leading to heart disease.

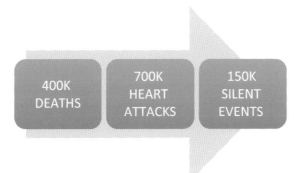

Figure 1.2 Cardiovascular disease in the US claims one in six lives each year.

deaths in the US today is attributable to CAD — every 34 seconds, one American will have a heart attack and every one minute, a person will die from the event.

Clearly, cardiovascular disease is a problem of epidemic proportions and must be addressed in more effective ways. We have the technology and tools to make diagnoses in more efficient ways and we are able to identify risk factors in younger adults. We must cultivate a culture of health rather than a culture of excess. It is clear that unhealthy habits and the development of risk factors for cardiovascular diseases begin early in life. In fact, a study published in *The Lancet*[5] in November 2013, reported a 25% increase in stroke rates in younger adults — aged 23–64 — that supports the need to intervene early. Stroke rates in patients under the age of 20 have increased significantly over the last ten years. The pathophysiology and risk for both stroke and heart disease are quite similar. This new study should serve as a wake up call for both healthcare professionals as well as young adults to become more engaged in prevention.

The fallout of heart disease

Heart disease can result in significant morbidity. Multiple myocardial infarctions (MI) can result in chronic congestive heart failure (CHF), recurrent hospitalizations and reduced quality of life. Moreover, depression amongst individuals suffering with chronic heart disease is significant and further contributes to exacerbations of heart failure and attacks of unstable angina. Heart disease can limit one's ability to work and socialize with family and friends. Those that suffer from heart disease are at increased risk for other chronic disease and more susceptible to infection and other severe illnesses. Ultimately, heart disease can result in sudden cardiac death. In many patients who have had a prior MI and have left ventricular dysfunction, the risk of ventricular fibrillation and sudden death is quite high — scar surrounding a prior infarct predisposes these patients to life-threatening arrhythmias. Although the survival rates for sudden cardiac death or cardiac arrest outside of the hospital are quite low, early defibrillation and the advent of implantable cardioverter-defibrillators (ICDs) have improved these rates significantly — but at what ultimate cost? In this era of healthcare reform in the US, we are beginning to look to prevention to

---

[5] Felgin, V. L., Forouzanfar, M. H., Krishnamurthi, R. *et al.* (2014). Global and regional burden of stroke during 1990–2010: findings from the Global Burden of Disease Study 2010. *The Lancet*, Volume 383, Issue 9913, 245–255.

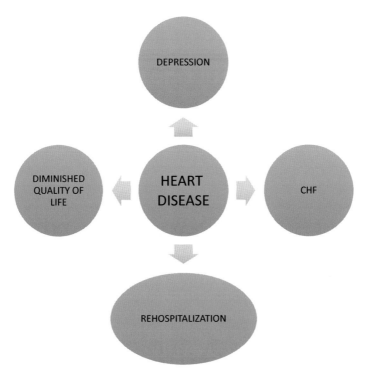

Figure 1.3   Fallout of heart disease.

help save lives and curtail expenditures. We must continue to develop new strategies that address risk factor modification in hopes of reducing the burden of disease worldwide. The costs to society are great — economically, heart disease and its complications continue to account for a great deal of financial healthcare expenditures both in the US and abroad.

Women and heart disease — Defining the scope of the problem

According to the American Heart Association nearly 1 in 3 women have some form of cardiovascular disease and, since 1984, deaths in females have greatly exceeded deaths in males. During this same time period, numerous advances in technology to treat heart disease (both acute and chronic) have evolved and resulted in substantial reductions in death. But interestingly in 2010, only 25% of CABG patients and only 32% of PCI patients were female. In 2011, only 32% of transplant patients were female. The dichotomy of equal prevalence and unequal treatment is perplexing and must be better understood in order for change to occur. The fact remains that heart disease in women continues to present a major public health problem — interventions must be made in order to reduce mortality and morbidity in women from cardiovascular disease in both the US and in Europe.

Chapter Two

Gender Differences in Disease Manifestation and Presentation

Men and women manifest chronic diseases in predictable ways. We are, of course, of the same species and composed of the same basic genetic materials; however, there are important differences that can change the way in which a disease may present and progress. Cardiovascular disease is the leading cause of death in both sexes but heart disease may develop in each gender in significantly different ways. Hormonal differences between men and women not only determine our outward appearances and gender-specific sexual development but may also have a significant impact on how our bodies are affected by certain risk factors and respond to a particular disease process. In addition, exogenous hormone therapies may also have a significant impact on how patients respond to a disease over time.

The best way to address the complex issue of gender-specific manifestations of heart disease (and response to therapy) is to break down the differences into several categories:

1. Structural Differences
2. Biologic/Hormonal Differences
3. Differences in Disease Progression
4. Differences in Response to Therapy and Outcomes

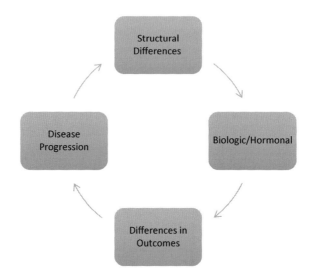

Figure 2.1   Factors affecting cardiovascular disease in women.

Structural differences

Although we share developmental and embryologic similarities, there are structural differences in the cardiovascular systems of men and women. The heart begins to form during week five of development and develops from splanchnic mesenchyme. When completely developed, women's hearts are smaller than men's. This is mainly a result of body size: a smaller body size equates to a proportionally smaller heart size. In addition, blood vessels in women are smaller. Hormones such as estrogen and progesterone promote development of smaller blood vessels (particularly coronary arteries) in women. Smaller blood vessels are more likely to form plaques that become unstable and rupture in the setting of an acute myocardial infarction. The smaller size of the coronary arteries results in more technically difficult angioplasty and stenting procedures. These smaller coronary arteries are more likely to tear or dissect during a percutaneous coronary intervention (PCI).

Biologic differences

Obviously there are significant biologic and hormonal differences between men and women. Although both men and women have some levels of all of the sex hormones — estrogen, progesterone, and testosterone — these levels are very different in each gender. Higher levels of estrogens and progesterone with lower levels of testosterone (commonly seen in most pre-menopausal females) can have a significant impact on the manifestations and progression of coronary artery disease. In men, elevated levels of testosterone promote the formation of larger coronary arteries and blood vessels. Women, in contrast, have higher levels of estrogen and progesterone and form smaller blood vessels. Estrogen has been shown to be protective for pre-menopausal women and reduces their risk of heart disease. However, the precipitous drop in estrogen levels at the time of menopause is associated with a significant increase risk for coronary events.

Differences in disease progression

Acute myocardial infarction occurs when there is a complete occlusion of a coronary artery. The acute closure of the artery most often occurs due to the rupture of a vulnerable plaque. These vulnerable plaques are made of fats, cholesterol and inflammatory cells called macrophages. Interestingly, these plaques appear to be biologically different in men versus women. In men, these plaques are often heavily calcified and hard. In contrast, many of these plaques in women tend to be a bit softer, less calcified and more prone to rupture.[1] Moreover, many women who suffer from acute myocardial infarction have no significant angiographically

---

[1] Bairey Merz, C. N., Shaw, L. J., Reis, S. E. *et al.* (2006). Insights from the NHLBI-sponsored WISE study, part II: gender differences in presentation, diagnosis, and outcome with regard to gender-based pathophysiology of atherosclerosis and macrovascular and microvascular coronary disease. *J Am Coll Cardiol*, Volume 47, S21–S29.

demonstrable disease at cardiac catheterization, but have evidence of plaque ulceration and rupture.[2] Many researchers postulate that the smaller size of women's coronary arteries may contribute to this type of non-obstructive plaque rupture. Women also tend to have more widespread disease, and disease that is less likely to be classified as high-grade obstructions; instead, they are more likely to have mild to moderately obstructive disease.[3] Studies have shown that patients with mild to moderately obstructive disease are prescribed evidence-based secondary prevention therapies at much lower rates than those with more significant obstructions.[4]

Differences in response to therapies and outcomes

We have discussed several structural and biologic/hormonal gender differences, as well as differences in disease progression, earlier in this chapter. In addition to these differences in disease manifestation, there are also gender differences in how patients may respond to therapy. Fortunately, today there are many evidence-based therapies for the treatment of heart disease. These therapies range from cardio-protective drugs, such as beta-blockers and ACE inhibitors, to cholesterol-lowering drugs, such as statins, and all have been shown to reduce mortality in appropriate patients. Certain drugs such as ACE inhibitors have been shown in a few clinical trials to have more profound effects in women as compared to men.[5] Moreover, certain drugs have different pharmacokinetics in women as compared to

---

[2] Reynolds, H. R., Srichai, M. B., Iqbal, S. N. *et al.* (2011) Mechanism of myocardial infarction in women without angiographically obstructive coronary artery disease. *Circulation*, Volume 124, 1414–1425.

[3] Smilowitz, N. R., Sampson, B. A., Abrecht, C. R. *et al.* (2011). Women have less severe and extensive coronary atherosclerosis in fatal cases of ischemic heart disease: an autopsy study. *Am Heart J*, Volume 161, 681–688.

[4] Maddox, T. M., Ho, P. M., Dai, D. *et al.* (2010). Utilization of secondary prevention therapies in patients with nonobstructive coronary artery disease identified during cardiac catheterization. *Circ Cardiovasc Qual Outcomes*, Volume 3, 632–641.

[5] Seeland, U. and Regitz-Zagrosek, V. (2012). Sex and gender differences in cardiovascular drug therapy. *Handb Exp Pharmacol*, Volume 214, 211–236.

men and require careful dose adjustment. Studies have shown that certain drug combinations are associated with better outcomes in women, particularly beta-blocker/diuretic combination therapies.[6] Healthcare providers must be aware of which combinations are most efficacious for our patients and ensure that women are treated with the appropriate evidence-based medications.

As previously mentioned, many women do not seem to receive the same aggressive treatments for heart disease as compared to men. The data clearly supports an early invasive approach in patients with acute ST-segment myocardial infarction with a goal of prompt revascularization. In cases of non-ST-elevation myocardial intarction (NSTEMI), higher-risk patients (those with a positive troponin) also benefit from an early invasive approach. While all invasive cardiac procedures are associated with a finite risk for complication, men seem to experience fewer complications than their female counterparts. Many clinicians are more reluctant to send women to invasive procedures because of the fact that they have been shown to have higher complication rates; this is despite the fact that overall outcomes are improved with this strategy. In women undergoing cardiac catheterization and revascularization, bleeding and adverse vascular events requiring transfusion or intervention are more common.[7-9] These adverse events can range from bleeding and femoral hematomas to vascular compromise requiring surgical repair. Many of these complications can lead to prolonged hospitalization

---

[6]Wassertheil-Smoller, S., Psaty, B., Greenland, P. *et al.* (2004). Association between cardiovascular outcomes and antihypertensive drug treatment in older women. *JAMA*, Volume 292(23), 2849–2859.

[7]Peterson, E. D., Lansky, A. J., Kramer, J. *et al.* (2001). Effect of gender on the outcomes of contemporary percutaneous coronary intervention. *Am J Cardiol*, Volume 88, 359–364.

[8]Argulian, E., Patel, A. D., Abramson, J. L. *et al.* (2006). Gender differences in short-term cardiovascular outcomes after percutaneous coronary interventions. *Am J Cardiol*, Volume 98, 48–53.

[9]Tavris, D. R., Gallauresi, B. A., Dey, S. *et al.* (2007). Risk of local adverse events by gender following cardiac catheterization. *Pharmacoepidemiol Drug Saf*, Volume 16, 125–131.

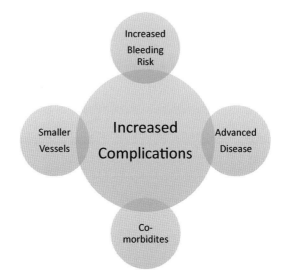

Figure 2.2 Factors associated with higher complication rates in women.

and longer recovery times. However, more recent studies have shown that while women continue to have higher complication rates with cardiac catheterization and intervention, these rates are declining.[10] One possible explanation for the reduction in complication rates in women may be the increasing use of radial access techniques (as opposed to the traditional femoral approach) in women over the last decade. A comparison of women undergoing cardiac catheterization and revascularization via femoral versus radial techniques has shown a significant decrease in procedure-related complication rates in women who were accessed via the radial approach.[11]

[10]Ahmed, B., Piper, W. D., Malenka, D. *et al.* (2009). Significantly improved vascular complications among women undergoing percutaneous coronary intervention: a report from the Northern New England Percutaneous Coronary Intervention Registry. *Circulation*, Volume 2, 423–429.

[11]Pristipino, C., Pelliccia, F., Granatelli, A. *et al.* (2007). Comparison of access-related bleeding complications in women versus men undergoing percutaneous coronary catheterization using the radial versus femoral artery. *Am J Cardiol*, Volume 99(9), 1216–1221.

The trend toward higher complications for women is also noted in women undergoing coronary artery bypass grafting (CABG). As compared to men, women have higher rates of morbidity and mortality with CABG.[12] There are many reasons that may explain these findings including the fact that women often present for revascularization surgery with more co-morbidities, or more advanced disease. Women also were found to have more diabetes, more hypertension and pre-existing cerebro-vascular disease. In addition, from a technical aspect, women tended to have less available arterial grafts and their procedures were more often determined to be urgent or emergent. Overall, both peri-operative and post-operative cardiac and neurologic complications are higher in women as compared to men.[13]

We are fortunate to have many advanced therapies to treat heart disease in the modern era. These therapies have been proven in large clinical trials to reduce mortality and improve outcome. Female patients account for a significant proportion of cardiovascular events yet treatments and outcomes often differ from those in males. Disease presentation and progression is affected by numerous gender-specific factors and can impact the effectiveness of our available therapies. In order to improve outcomes in women, we must continue to apply data-driven therapies to both sexes, but with a better understanding of the biologic, hormonal and structural factors that may affect they way in which patients may respond.

[12]Woods, S. E., Noble, G., Smith, J. M. *et al.* (2003). The influence of gender in patients undergoing coronary artery bypass graft surgery: an eight-year prospective hospitalized cohort study. *Journal of the American College of Surgeons*, Volume 196(3), 428–434.

[13]Hogue, C. W., Sundt, T. III, Barzilai, B. *et al.* (2001). Cardiac and neurologic complications identify risks for mortality for both men and women undergoing coronary artery bypass graft surgery. *Anesthesiology*, Volume 95(5), 1074–1078.

Chapter Three

Gender Differences in Testing and Evaluation

The diagnosis of coronary artery disease can be challenging. Gender differences in patient presentation and biological differences in the extent and in the progression of cardiovascular disease make the evaluation of risk in women even more complex. While men are more likely to have discrete lesions within the coronary arteries, angiographic studies have shown that women have more diffuse disease — these types of abnormalities are much harder to detect on routine testing. However, one study has demonstrated that when women do have typical symptoms, they are more likely to have more significant, life-threatening disease. Moreover, it has been shown that over the last several decades, mortality from heart attack is much higher in women than in men. These higher cardiovascular disease mortality rates makes early detection and prevention an even more pressing matter in women as compared to men. Unfortunately, routine testing and, even more concerning, follow-up testing, is less likely to be applied in women as compared to men.

When approaching a patient suspected of having coronary artery disease, healthcare providers must approach both sexes equally. Although it is vital to understand and incorporate gender differences into formulating plans for evaluation, we must consider the fact that women are in fact undertreated and underserved. From a clinical standpoint, physicians must evaluate risk factors (in both sexes) and develop a pre-test probability for the presence or absence of disease. Pre-test probabilities are defined as the subjective likelihood of the presence of a disease prior to diagnostic testing. Properly predicting the pre-test probability of disease is integral to choosing the proper diagnostic testing strategy. It is important to consider the use of Bayes' theorem for determining the appropriate testing and workup of a woman presenting with possible coronary artery disease.[1] By applying Bayes' principles, we are able to select the best test for evaluating a particular female patient — providing the highest possible yield while at the same time limiting false positive results.

Another important factor in choosing and successfully performing a diagnostic test is determining the prevalence of the disease. Prevalence is defined as the proportion of the population found to have the disease. Younger women typically have a low prevalence of coronary artery disease and tend to present later in life with more severe disease.

However, some testing can be more accurate in men when compared to women. For instance, some types of exams, such as exercise stress testing, yield higher rates of false negative results in women. Further compounding this issue is the fact that women who have symptoms of heart disease are less likely to be referred for further diagnostic testing.[2]

In the US today, exercise stress testing is the most common and most cost-effective screening test for the evaluation for

---

[1] Rifkin, R. D. and Hood, W. B. Jr. (1977). Bayesian analysis of electrocardiographic exercise stress testing. *N Engl J Med*, Volume 297, 681–686.
[2] Daugherty, S. L., Peterson, P. N., Magid, D. J. *et al.* (2008). The relationship between gender and clinical management after exercise stress testing. *Am Heart J*, Volume 156, 301–307.

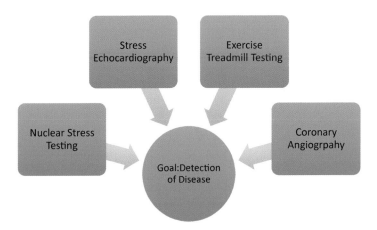

Figure 3.1 Detection of cardiovascular disease: testing options.

coronary artery disease in both men and women.[3] In women who have an intermediate pre-test probability of coronary artery disease the American College of Cardiology recommends the addition of imaging such as either echocardiography or nuclear SPECT to exercise stress testing in order to improve yield. However, these imaging tests tend to be a bit less accurate in women as compared to men. For instance, nuclear stress testing in women tends to produce more false positives due to breast attenuation defects that can be mistaken for areas of myocardial ischemia. In addition, the size of the left ventricular cavity is smaller in women and the coronary arteries tend to be smaller in women as compared to men and both of these factors make SPECT stress testing less accurate. Exercise echocardiography can also be useful in detecting coronary artery disease in women. However, due to body habitus, acoustic windows for obtaining adequate images for interpretation are often more limited in

---

[3] Cohen, M. C., Stafford, R. S. and Misra, B. (1999). Stress testing: national patterns and predictors of test ordering. *Am Heart J*, Volume 138, 1019–1024.

women. When a meta-analysis was performed comparing the accuracy of nuclear SPECT versus stress echocardiography imaging in women, no difference was found. The sensitivity and specificity of both methods were comparable in women yet, when compared to men, there were more false positives.[4] Importantly, in another study, women with no evidence of electrocardiography (EKG) or echocardiographic abnormalities during stress testing had a remarkable cardiac event free survival (>96%). In contrast, women with abnormalities and evidence of ischemia have a very high event rate and event free survival is much lower (<55%).[5]

As with most diagnostic testing, there are risks to the patient associated with each modality that must be considered when choosing appropriate diagnostic testing. These exposure risks are actually different in men and women with women requiring higher doses in order to produce similar image quality. With nuclear SPECT imaging and cardiac CT scanning there are finite risks associated with radiation exposure. The most common radioisotope utilized for stress testing is technetium-99m (Myoview). In the stress test protocol women receive 10.57 mSv (millisieverts) versus 8.81 mSv for men. The Health Physics Society estimates that exposures below 500 mSv most often have no visible effects at the time of the exposure. To put this in perspective, all of us receive "background radiation" exposure annually in the amount of 4 mSv — therefore, a stress test accounts for the equivalent of nearly three years of background radiation exposure. CT scanning accounts for higher radiation doses than SPECT imaging. The doses of radiation that we

[4] Grady, D., Chaput, L. and Kristof, M. (2003). Diagnosis and treatment of coronary heart disease in women: systematic reviews of evidence on selected topics: evidence report/technology assessment No. 81 (prepared by the University of California, San Francisco–Stanford Evidence-Based Practice Center under contract No. 290-97-0013). Stanford Evidence-Based Practice Center. AHRQ publication No. 03-E037.
[5] Heupler, S., Mehta, R., Lobo, A. *et al.* (1997). Prognostic implications of exercise echocardiography in women with known or suspected coronary artery disease. *J Am Coll Cardiol*, Volume 30, 414–420.

receive are cumulative and risks increase over time. In the US alone, it is estimated that nearly 2% of cancers are due to radiation exposures during diagnostic testing.[6] Radiation exposure has been associated with the development of certain types of cancers including lymphomas and certain types of leukemias. When evaluating women of childbearing age it is important to ensure that they are not pregnant before undertaking a test that involves radiation exposure.

What's the best way to evaluate women for heart disease?

The American College of Cardiology (ACC) has produced an algorithm for the evaluation of heart disease in women. Based on the best available data, the recommended approach is as follows: initial evaluation must consist of an assessment of risk factors and symptoms. Once the initial evaluation is performed, women should be divided into two categories — those with symptoms and those without symptoms. In asymptomatic women, no stress testing is recommended unless there are other high-risk features such as significant family history of premature heart disease, or a combination of several other traditional risk factors. The ACC recommends further that the initial test of choice should be an exercise EKG test — unless there are issues that may preclude interpretation, such as a left bundle branch block or the inability to adequately exercise to the appropriate level on the treadmill. In fact, the pre-test probability of finding coronary artery disease in asymptomatic women without significant risk factors (in all age groups) is quite low. In contrast, women who have symptoms require much more comprehensive evaluation. Even in women aged 30–60 with classic symptoms of angina, the pre-test probabilities are intermediate. However, in

---

[6]Mathews, J. D., Forsythe, A. V., Brady, Z. *et al.* (2013). Cancer risk in 680 000 people exposed to computed tomography scans in childhood or adolescence: data linkage study of 11 million Australians. *BMJ*, Volume 346, f2360. doi: 10.1136/bmj.f2360.

those who are older than 60 with classic symptoms, the pre-test probabilities are quite high for coronary artery disease. Moreover, women with atypical symptoms whom are older than 50 also have an intermediate-to-high-risk pre-test probability of having disease.

According to the ACC, in women with symptoms and normal baseline EKG (along with the ability to exercise) the exercise treadmill test is the test of choice. The Duke Activity Index is a questionnaire that can be used to determine if a potential patient will be able to adequately exercise during a treadmill test.[7, 8] If the functional capacity is determined to be less than 5 METS (metabolic equivalent of tasks), then a pharmacologic test is indicated. If an exercise stress test is negative, the negative predictive value for coronary artery disease is quite

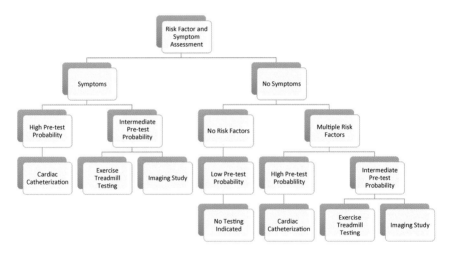

Figure 3.2   Proposed algorithm for the evaluation of heart disease in women.

[7]Bairey Merz, C. N., Olson, M., McGorray, S. *et al.* (2000). Physical activity and functional capacity measurement in women: a report from the NHLBI-sponsored WISE study. *J Womens Health Gend Based Med*, Volume 9, 769–777.

[8]Shaw, L. J., Olson, M. B., Kip, K. *et al.* The value of estimated functional capacity in estimating outcome: results from the NHLBI-sponsored Women's Ischemia Syndrome Evaluation (WISE) study. *J Am Coll Cardiol*, Volume 47, S36–S43.

low. However, if the test is inconclusive or positive in any way, further evaluation with either imaging-based testing or angiography is immediately indicated. A negative stress test with imaging will essentially rule out the presence of coronary artery disease in the majority of cases. Unfortunately, many women do not receive the comprehensive evaluation, screening and testing that is outlined above. In many cases, asymptomatic women with risk factors or women with atypical symptoms and risk factors are often not even evaluated with the indicated EKG and/ or EKG exercise stress testing. Moreover, many women who are evaluated and found to have indeterminate results are not sent along for further evaluation with either an imaging stress test or coronary angiography. These lapses in the diagnostic workup then leads to many preventable cardiac events in women.

Appropriate diagnostic testing is critical in the diagnosis and treatment of coronary artery disease. Making the proper data-driven choices when evaluating a patient with suspected heart disease can result in the prevention of devastating cardiac events. In women, diagnostic testing can provide additional challenges and some tests are not as accurate in women as they are in men. In addition, there are risks associated with each type of test and typical radiation exposures are higher in women as compared to men. Issues of fertility and pregnancy must also be considered when choosing a diagnostic approach. However, an organized algorithmic approach to the evaluation of heart disease in women can result in high diagnostic yields and proper treatment afforded to female patients at earlier stages of disease. Ultimately, timely diagnosis and treatment is likely to reduce the rate of death from heart disease in women both in the US and throughout the world.

Chapter Four

Gender Differences in the Treatment of Coronary Artery Disease

Women with coronary artery disease are undertreated and underserved. In the US alone approximately 16.8 million people have heart disease — of these 8.1 million are female. In previous chapters, we have discussed the ways in which heart disease presents differently (both biologically and clinically) in men and women. The data is clear that more women than men die from heart disease. Surprisingly to many, women's mortality rates due to heart disease are four to six times higher than from breast cancer. Women who present with myocardial infarction are more likely to have more complicated hospital courses and have a significantly higher mortality as compared to their male cohorts.[1] In fact, women presenting with cardiovascular disease are often misdiagnosed and

---

[1] Gharacholou, S. M., Alexander, K. P., Chen, A. Y. *et al.* (2010). Implications and reasons for the lack of use of reperfusion therapy in patients with ST-segment elevation myocardial infarction: findings from the CRUSADE initiative. *Am Heart J,* Volume 159, 757–763.

more likely to die from their first cardiac event.[2] In the CRUSADE trial it was found that approximately 30% of patients presenting with ST-elevation myocardial infarction (STEMI) were women and female sex was an independent predictor of failure to receive prompt reperfusion therapy even though the data supports early revascularization in STEMI patients.[1] In other clinical trials, women were found to present later, have longer door-to-balloon times, longer door-to-fibrinolysis times and were less likely to be treated with aspirin and beta-blockers within 24 hours of presentation.[3] It is clear that there is a significant gender gap in the care of an acute coronary syndromes — this gap must be addressed in order to improve the mortality rates in women with cardiovascular disease. Unless we recognize the problem and begin to educate ourselves, our colleagues and our patients, little will be done to impact survival rates of women with heart disease.

To impact change, we must all have a better understanding of why there is a dichotomy in cardiac care between men and women in the first place — certainly disease presentation plays a significant role. In addition, there is an erroneous public perception that heart disease is predominantly a disease of men. In order to understand why we see some differences in disease presentation and why public perception of the demographics of the disease is flawed we must again consider biological differences in men and women. As discussed in previous chapters, women often present with more diffuse coronary artery disease, more atypical symptoms and often present much later in the course of their illness. Women are affected differently by risk factors — for instance, women with diabetes are more

---

[2] Kudenchuk, P. J., Maynard, C., Martin, J. S. *et al.* (1996). Comparison of presentation, treatment, and outcome of acute myocardial infarction in men versus women (the Myocardial Infarction Triage and Intervention Registry). *Am J Cardiol*, Volume 78, 9–14.

[3] Subherwal, S., Bach, R. G., Chen, A. Y. *et al.* (2009). Baseline risk of major bleeding in non-ST-segment-elevation myocardial infarction: the CRUSADE (Can Rapid risk stratification of unstable angina patients suppress adverse outcomes with early implementation of the ACC/AHA Guidelines) Bleeding Score. *Circulation*, Volume 119, 1873–1882.

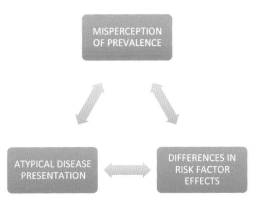

Figure 4.1 Biologic factors contributing to disparities in cardiovascular care in women.

likely to develop heart disease than men. In addition, cholesterol abnormalities such as low HDL (high-density lipoprotein) in women confer a much higher risk for the development of coronary artery disease. In women, hyperlipidemia, in particular LDL (low-density lipoprotein) abnormalities, seem to peak a decade later than men (around age 65) but a meta-analysis showed an increased risk of heart disease in women younger than 65 who do have elevated lipids, as compared to men with similar elevations.[4]

Evidence from numerous clinical trials over the last several decades has made the evaluation and treatment of acute coronary syndrome (ACS), including both non-ST-elevation myocardial infarction (NSTEMI) as well as STEMI quite clear.[5,6] The American

[4]Manolio, T. A., Pearson, T. A., Wenger, N. K. *et al.* (1992). Cholesterol and heart disease in older persons and women. Review of an NHLBI workshop. *Ann Epidemiol.* Volume 2, 161–176.

[5]O'Gara, P. T., Kushner, F. G., Ascheim, D. D. *et al.* (2013). ACCF/AHA Guideline for the Management of ST-Elevation Myocardial Infarction: A Report of the American College of Cardiology Foundation/American Heart Association Task Force on Practice Guidelines. *J Am Coll Cardiol.* Volume 61(4), e78–e140.

[6]2011 Writing Group Members, Wright, R. S., Anderson, J. L., Adams, C. D. *et al.* (2011). ACCF/AHA Focused update of the guidelines for the management of patients with unstable angina/non-ST-elevation myocardial infarction (updating the 2007 guideline). *Circulation*, Volume 123, 2022–2060.

College of Cardiology has developed guidelines that are well supported by the best available evidence. In NSTEMI and unstable
angina, expert consensus recommends an early invasive strategy in
high-risk patients — those with positive biomarkers and those with
any hemodynamic instability or refractory chest pain. In the setting
of STEMI, experts recommend prompt revascularization via primary
percutaneous coronary intervention (PCI) in PCI-capable facilities.
In the case of STEMI in a facility not capable of PCI, either thrombolytic therapy or rapid transfer to a PCI-ready facility is recommended.
Obviously, treatment with aspirin, beta-blockers, nitrates and anticoagulation with heparin, enoxaparin as well as the addition of
glycoprotein IIb/IIIa inhibitors is indicated in cases of NSTEMI as
well as peri-PCI in STEMI cases undergoing revascularization.

Most emergency departments and emergency management
systems (EMS) have well-established protocols in place for the pre-
hospital management of potential ACS patients. These protocols
are aimed at reducing delays in diagnosis and treatment. While not
every hospital is PCI-capable, there are significant increases in
mortality associated with delays in treatment after arrival to the
hospital.[7] Many EMS providers are able to transmit real-time EKG
tracings to ER physicians for rapid interpretation. There is a growing body of evidence to support pre-hospital administration of
thrombolytic therapy when transporting a patient to a non-PCI
capable hospital if a qualified EMS team and physician are able to
effectively communicate during the process of evaluation and
treatment.[8] On arrival to the emergency department, treatment
decisions are more rapidly made when pre-hospital care is initiated
in indicated patients. Research has proven that prompt diagnosis
and treatment is critical.

---

[7] Rathore, S. S., Curtis, J. P., Chen, J. *et al.* (2009). Association of door-to-balloon
time and mortality in patients admitted to hospital with ST elevation myocardial
infarction: national cohort study. *BMJ*, Volume 338, b1807.
[8] Roth, A., Barbash, G. I., Hod, H. *et al.* (1990). Should thrombolytic therapy be
administered in the mobile intensive care unit in patients with evolving myocardial
infarction? A pilot study. *J Am Coll Cardiol*, Volume 15, 932–936.

Over the last 20 years, advances in both the medical and early invasive strategies to treat ACS have resulted in significant reductions in mortality in men. However, in women rates of death from ACS and cardiovascular disease continue to either level off or continue to rise.[9] There is accumulating evidence that suggests that early intervention and revascularization in patients with NSTEMI reduces rates of subsequent cardiac events and death. However, there is also data that complication rates (particularly bleeding risks) in the setting of acute intervention are higher in women as compared to men. Adding to the difficulty in treating women, the presenting EKG in the emergency department is much less likely to be diagnostic and more women present with NSTEMI and ST depression than with classic STEMI. Biomarkers, a cornerstone in diagnosis and prognosis in myocardial infarction, also appear to be less often elevated in women on initial presentation.[10] We know that the presence of an elevated troponin in a NSTEMI is a hallmark for worse prognosis in both sexes and argues for a more aggressive, invasive approach to therapy. However, women with positive biomarkers often are not treated with the recommended early invasive strategy due to concerns over increased bleeding and complication rates.

The higher mortality rates in women with heart disease is fact — not just perception. Data from multiple registries and several retrospective studies have shown that women are not treated as aggressively as men. Women undergo less angiography and fewer coronary artery bypass grafting (CABG) procedures.[11] In fact, even women with documented heart disease and subse-

---

[9]Elsaesser, A. and Hamm, C. W. (2004). Acute coronary syndrome: the risk of being female. *Circulation*, Volume 109, 565–567.

[10]Wu, A. H. B., Apple, F. S., Gibler, W. B. *et al.* (1999). National Academy of Clinical Biochemistry Standards of Laboratory Practice: Recommendations for the use of cardiac markers in coronary artery diseases. *Clin Chem*, Volume 45, 1104–1121.

[11]Anand, S. S., Xie, C., Mehta, S. *et al.* (2005). Differences in the management and prognosis of women and men who suffer from acute coronary syndromes. *J Am Coll Cardiol*, Volume 46(10), 1845–1851.

quent cardiac events are much less likely to receive thrombolytic therapy and undergo invasive procedures such as coronary angiography and revascularization as compared to men.[12] In addition, women who do have invasive procedures tend to have higher complication rates.[13] Women who do undergo an invasive strategy are found to have smaller coronary arteries, more diffuse and widespread disease. Early data from *Circulation* in 1993 demonstrated that women undergoing CABG procedures have excess mortality and most of this is due to heart failure, smaller coronary arteries and fewer left internal mammary (LIMA) grafts.[14]

In a large meta-analysis conducted by the Agency for Healthcare Research and Policy (AHRQ) randomized controlled trials from 2001 to 2011 that compared treatment strategies and sex-specific differences were evaluated.[15] The purpose of the analysis was to examine treatment strategies in the setting of acute myocardial infarction in both men and women and compare results. The findings were quite powerful. In women presenting with an acute STEMI an early, aggressive invasive strategy with cardiac catheterization and PCI was far superior to fibrinolysis in reducing further cardiovascular events. In addition, the study also found a trend that in women with unstable angina, an early invasive strategy was also superior in reducing future events. Most significantly, the analysis also found that when comparing revas-

[12]Weitzman, S., Cooper, L., Chambless, L. *et al.* (1997). Gender, racial, and geographic differences in the performance of cardiac diagnostic and therapeutic procedures for the hospitalized acute myocardial infraction in four states. *Am J Cardiol,* Volume 79, 722–726.

[13]Johnstone, N., Schenck-Gustafsson, K. and Lagerqvist, B. (2011). Are we suing cardiovascular medications and coronary angiography appropriately in men and women with chest pain? *European Heart J*, Volume 32, 1331–1336.

[14]O'Connor, G. T., Morton, J. R., Diehl, M. J. *et al.* (1993). Differences between men and women in hospital mortality associated with coronary bypass graft surgery. *Circulation*, Volume 88, 2104–2110.

[15]Dolor, R. J., Melloni, C., Chatterjee, R. *et al.* (2012). Treatment strategies for women with coronary artery disease. Rockville (MD): Agency for Healthcare Research and Quality (US); 2012 Aug. Comparative Effectiveness Reviews, No. 66.

cularization to conservative medical therapy in women the invasive strategy was associated with improved outcomes. By contrast, the outcomes and event rate for either treatment strategy was similar in male patients. However, in spite of these findings men continue to be treated more aggressively and more often with an early invasive approach, as compared to women presenting in similar fashion.

Not only are women treated differently when presenting with an acute event, evidence suggests that they are also treated differently during the recovery period after an acute cardiac event and at discharge. Some studies indicate that guideline-based therapies are not equally applied in men and women. Even more disturbing is the fact that women who are discharged after acute myocardial infarction are less likely to be prescribed appropriate, evidence-based medications, such as aspirin, ACE inhibitors, beta-blockers and cholesterol-lowering agents. These women have been shown to have higher rates of re-hospitalization and debilitating refractory ischemia. In fact, women, particularly if older, Hispanic or African American are even less likely to receive these evidence-based medications that have been shown to confer mortality benefits in major clinical trials.

Although we have long been aware that post-event counseling and lifestyle modification has been associated with decreased rates of subsequent events, women also seem to receive much less pre-discharge counseling. When treating women with ACS, there seems to be less focus on risk factor modification, lifestyle changes and secondary prevention as compared to men. Data from numerous studies have shown that in women presenting with ACS the rates of obesity, hypertension, hypercholesterolemia and obesity are much higher than in men.[16] Only smoking is more prevalent in men with heart disease. However, smoking is a major risk factor

---

[16]Shehab, A., Yasin, J., Hashim, M. J. *et al.* (2012). Gender differences in acute coronary syndrome in Arab Emirati women — implications for clinical management. *Angiology*, Volume 64(1), 9–14.

for women as well and in women presenting with ACS that are under the age of 50 nearly 60% of these events are attributable to tobacco abuse. There is good evidence to suggest that *all* women with coronary artery disease benefit from smoking cessation.[17] Interestingly, studies show that women tend to have more difficulty with smoking cessation than men and without treatment and counseling are more likely to relapse and begin smoking again. Yet with all these increased modifiable risk factors, women continue to receive fewer interventions aimed at secondary prevention even prior to discharge from the hospital following an acute cardiac event. In a study examining risk factor modification and outcome after ACS, researchers found that women were less likely to achieve target blood pressure, lipids and blood sugars over a six-year follow-up period.[18] Clearly, as a whole, we are doing a very poor job in treating women after an acute cardiac event. We have many missed opportunities for intervention and secondary prevention.

An important component to the effective treatment of coronary artery disease is the outpatient care in the months to years following an acute event. As discussed above, risk factor modification and lifestyle changes are very important in both men and women. In addition, cardiac rehabilitation can be an important part of recovery. Unfortunately, women are not as likely to be referred to cardiac rehabilitation (as compared to men) and are less likely to participate in organized rehabilitation activities.[19] One study in particular found that recovery goals differed significantly between the sexes and may explain some of the differences in rehabilitation

---

[17]Kawachi, I., Colditz, M. B., Stampfer, M. J. *et al.* (1994). Smoking cessation and time course of decreased risks of coronary heart disease in middle-aged women. *Arch Intern Med*, Volume 154, 169–175.

[18]Reibis, R. K., Bestehorn, K., Pittrow, D. *et al.* (2009). Elevated risk profile of women in secondary prevention of coronary artery disease: a 6-year survey of 117,913 patients. *J Womens Health (Larchmt)*, Volume 18(8), 1123–1131.

[19]Grande, G. and Romppel, M. (2011). Gender differences in recovery goals in patients after acute myocardial infarction. *J Cardiopulm Rehabil Prev*, Volume 31(3), 164–172.

participation. In this investigation, women placed higher importance on returning to household duties whereas men were more concerned with developing physical endurance and returning to work quickly.[20] Studies have shown that cardiac rehabilitation referral after an acute coronary event by physicians has been biased against the elderly and women in particular.[21] Cardiac rehabilitation has been associated with improved outcomes and is an essential part of recovery after myocardial infarction and in particular CABG procedures.[22] It has further been proven that patients who either do not attend or attend rehab sessions less than 25% of the time have more than double the mortality rate of those with more regular attendance.[23] In addition, participation in rehabilitation programs is associated with a much higher rate of smoking cessation in cardiac patients — an essential part of secondary prevention.[24] Yet again, we miss these secondary prevention opportunities with our female patients.

We have clear evidence for the most effective treatments for ACS and coronary artery disease that is based on many years of work and several very large randomized controlled clinical trials. We also have a growing body of evidence for post-cardiac-event interventions including risk factor modification and lifestyle changes that clearly result in decreased mortality and reduction in subsequent events. However, the evidence suggests that women

---

[20] *Ibid.*

[21] Cottin, Y., Cambou, J. P., Cassilas, J. M. *et al.* (2004). Specific profile and referral bias of rehabilitated patients after an acute coronary syndrome. *J Cardiopulm Rehabil*, Volume 24(1), 38–44.

[22] Pack, Q. R., Goel, K., Lahr, B. D. *et al.* (2013). Participation in cardiac rehabilitation and survival following coronary artery bypass graft surgery: a community based study. *Circulation*, Volume 128, 590–597.

[23] Beauchamp, A., Worcester, M. Ng, A. *et al.* (2013). Attendance at cardiac rehabilitation is associated with lower all-cause mortality after 14 years of follow-up. *Heart*, Volume 99, 620–625.

[24] Dawood, N., Vaccarino, V., Reid, K. J. *et al.* (2008). Predictors of Smoking Cessation After a Myocardial Infarction: The Role of Institutional Smoking Cessation Programs in Improving Success. *Arch Intern Med*, Volume 168(18), 1961–1967.

are not treated as aggressively as men in the acute setting and fewer interventions are made in the post-event period as well. Ultimately, we are missing the mark in treating women — we must apply the same guidelines and standards of care to both sexes in order to achieve more equitable outcomes.

Chapter Five

Exploring the Root Causes

It is very clear that women with heart disease are not receiving the same care as men. We continue to fall short in diagnosis, testing and treatment of women with coronary artery disease (CAD). As mentioned previously, mortality rates for men continue to decline while those for women continue to stay the same (and in some cases increase slightly). In previous chapters we have considered the biological differences in disease presentation and progression. In addition, we have discussed the atypical symptoms that women often experience and the fact that some diagnostic tests are not as accurate in women. This makes diagnosis more challenging for even experienced providers with the best of intentions. Over the last several decades we have amassed a great deal of evidence for the best approach to treating acute myocardial infarction and unstable angina. Now, more than ever, we have multiple potentially life-saving therapies at our disposal when treating cardiac events. A review of the literature supports the fact that evidence-based therapies and clinical guidelines are not applied equally in men and women.

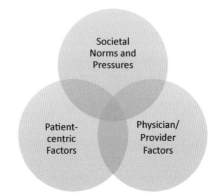

Figure 5.1   Factors affecting gender disparities in cardiovascular care.

Why exactly is this? What are the root causes for the phenomenon gender inequality? More importantly, what can we do about it?

In order to best answer these questions, we must first explore gender roles in the US and the UK — what they have been in the past, and how they are changing as our governments and economies evolve. The way in which society perceives individual genders may very well have a significant impact on how and why women receive different care when it comes to heart disease.

Television programs set in the 1950s and 1960s depicted the doting housewife, caring for the children at home while the man of the house goes off to work in his suit and tie. In the US today, the stereotypical 1950s housewife is a rare occurrence. In general, gender roles are norms that are defined by society — but this definition does not mean that these are the only *acceptable* roles. In the US and the UK, traditional gender roles have been associated with more aggression and dominance in men, and more passivity and nurturing behaviors in women. Things are changing — in a study released in May 2013 by the Pew Research Center, 40% of women were found to serve as the leading breadwinners for the family. This is in stark contrast to 11% in 1960. Of these breadwinner women, 40% are married and have higher incomes than their male spouses. Even with more women working outside the home, the traditional stereotypes of women as the primary homemaker places additional pressure and responsibilities on working mothers. In many cases, they continue to provide meals, assist with homework and provide most of the direct childcare and child management needs. Studies support the fact that women are the primary reason that other family members seek out healthcare. They ensure that appointments are made and attended for both children and spouse. Career-minded, successful women often find that there are not enough hours in the day to perform well in high-level jobs as well as excel as a wife and mother. Ultimately, something has to give — and often it is the busy mother's health.

Studies have shown that working mothers with children at home experience more stress and actually secrete higher levels of cortisol as compared to unemployed women.[1] This response is independent of whether they are married or not — having a spouse and working as a mom makes no difference in stress levels. Interestingly, the cortisol levels seemed to rise throughout the workday and no decline was seen once at home. Women have been found to have higher blood pressure as occupational status and work skill increases.[2] Other investigations have documented differences in the ways in which stress hormones such as catecholamines rise and fall during the day for working women versus working men. In men in management positions, levels of epinephrine and norepinephrine were seen to peak during the workday and sharply decline once they arrived home.[3] In contrast, female managers were found to have levels of catecholamines that increased throughout the workday and

---

[1] Leucken, L. J., Suarez, E. C., Kuhn, C. M. *et al.* (1997). Stress in employed women: impact of marital status and children at home on neurohormone output and home strain. *Psychosom Med*, Volume 59, 352–359.

[2] Light, K. C., Turner, J. R. and Hinderliter, A. L. (1992). Job strain and ambulatory work blood pressure in healthy young men and women. *Hypertension*, Volume 20, 214–218.

[3] Frankenhaeuser, M., Lundberg, U., Frederickson, M. *et al.* (1989). Stress on and off the job as related to sex and occupational status in white-collar workers. *J Organizational Behav*, Volume 10, 321–346.

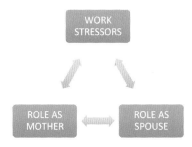

Figure 5.2   Cardiac stressors in women.

then continued to rise once arriving at home. Cortisol, and other catecholamines (stress hormones) are often associated with increased cardiovascular strain and cardiac events in those individuals with risk factors or who are predisposed to disease.

Stress levels alone at work are insufficient to explain the health consequences experienced by working women. It is more likely the complex interaction of multiple stressors related to the performance of multiple complex roles — work, wife and mother. Data from the Framingham database found a very strong correlation between CAD and employed women with multiple children.[4] It is clear that women experience different stressors than men and the biological and psychological responses to these stressors can be quite variable. Moreover, coping with the challenges of multiple roles and the pressures of societal norms can be challenging. Gender disparities in care for heart disease may be due to a combination of factors; some physician/provider centric and others that are more patient centered. These "root causes" cannot easily be explained nor are they easily corrected.

Often, in situations where we see multi-factorial causes for complex problems, it is helpful to separate possible etiologies into

[4] Haynes, S. G. and Feinleib, M. (1982). Women, work, and coronary heart disease: Results from the Framingham 10-year follow-up study. In Berman, P. and Ramey, E. (eds), *Women: A Developmental Perspective* (NIH Publication No. 82:2298). Washington, DC, US Government Printing Office.

individual parts. In exploring the root causes for gender disparities in cardiac care, we must consider patient-related factors, societal pressures/factors as well as physician and healthcare system related factors.

Patient-centric causes

It is clear that women often have different stressors than men. The data supports the idea that women who work feel a profound pressure to excel at all aspects of life: mother, professional and wife. Many women feel that in order to attain success, she must put others' needs ahead of her own. Even in women who do not work outside the home but are homemakers who care for children and support a spouse in his career, there is often a lack of attention paid to their own needs. Women seek out less care than men and often present much later in the course of their disease. Often, women do not take the time to work on risk factor modification and continue with negative health habits.

In many families it is the mother who makes sure that the children have all of their preventative health appointments and regular physical exams. The mother makes sure that the children have received any medications and tests that they may need. Often, the female spouse is involved in making sure that her male spouse makes and attends his preventative healthcare appointments. Moreover, if lifestyle changes must be made — such as changes in diet and exercise — it is often the wife who makes sure that the husband is able to comply. When women spend so much time advocating for others — children and spouse — their own needs often are forgotten. By the time a busy wife and mother has finished a day's work, prepared dinner and cared for the family, exercise and time focused on her own health is not a priority.

In many families in the modern era, males have taken on larger roles in caregiving for children as well as in meal preparation and other household duties. Marriage in the US and the UK today is much more of a partnership — this is in stark contrast to the 1950s stereotype. However, women continue to experience more stress at home as compared to men. Given the extreme pressure that women feel to excel and to provide for the needs of the family, it is common to see anxiety and depression in many professional women. The development of depression and anxiety can further complicate her ability to take control of her own healthcare and make healthy lifestyle choices.

It is clear that one specific reason why women may not seek out care may very well be that they are absolutely overwhelmed by multiple roles. Men deal with professional stressors but seem to be able to relax once at home. In contrast, women who work simply continue the stressful work associated with family life upon entering the home in the evening. The bottom line is that women feel that they do not have any time left for themselves. In order to excel at all roles — work, wife and mother — no time is left to focus on their own needs.

Societal pressures

Societal norms place an enormous pressure on women. In the US today, women are expected to be the primary caregiver for the children in the family and provide a pleasant home environment for her husband. Even though more women work outside the home than in past decades (and 40% are the primary breadwinners) pressures still exist. Some families have adapted remarkably well and the male spouse has begun to accept more of the family/childcare responsibilities — however, these are still in the minority. Women make up a significant proportion of the professional workforce, yet much of our society still expects the images of the 1950s household to continue. Television, movies, magazines and the mainstream media all contribute to the stereotype. Because of this ever-present and ubiquitous exposure to these images of "the perfect wife and mother", women experience societal pressures that men just do not face. These societal pressures are not without significant consequence. When there are issues in the home such as spousal infidelity or behavioral troubles with the children, many working/career women immediately blame themselves and the fact that they are attempting to manage both career and home life — a difficult (if not sometimes impossible) balance. This constant feeling of inadequacy can lead to depression as well as other health problems such as hypertension, obesity and type 2 diabetes.

The job of wife and mother leaves very little time for exercise, visits to the doctors and preventative care activities. As a result, obesity, high blood pressure and type 2 diabetes are common — many times these go unnoticed and untreated. Poor nutrition and a sedentary lifestyle become the norm.

Physician/provider factors

Physicians and providers often come to a patient encounter with preconceived notions that may introduce bias and affect their ability to make an accurate diagnosis. Unfortunately, when women present with atypical symptoms (as they often do), they may be quickly labeled as suffering from anxiety or depression. Often they are not properly evaluated for CAD at the time of the physician encounter and are quickly dismissed with an anxiolytic or anti-depressant. When clinicians are quick to make assumptions about a particular case, a complete history and physical exam is often never properly performed — adding to the chances of a missed diagnosis. In addition, even though there is scientific evidence to the contrary, many physicians continue to think of heart disease as a disease of men. When discussing preventative care with women, both doctor and patient tend to focus more on breast and gyneco-logical cancer screenings and often lose sight of screening for cardiovascular disease and its risk factors.

Women remain undertreated and underserved when it comes to heart disease. Yet, more women than men die of heart disease every single year. In order to successfully reverse this trend and ensure that women begin to get equal (and evidence-based) treatment we must carefully examine possible explanations for the dichotomy. There are no easy answers to this dilemma. As evidenced by the paucity of data on this subject we have yet to fully understand all of the root causes. For now, we must work to close the gender gap in care through a better understanding of the pressures that women face at home and at work. We must spend more time engaging with each patient during an office visit — we may only get one chance to make a difference and change the course of her disease.

Chapter Six

Closing the Gap: Strategies to Effect Change

We have seen in previous chapters that women are at significant risk for death from cardiovascular disease. Women remain undertreated and underserved. More women than men die of heart disease every year. Women tend to present with more severe disease, more advanced disease and have more negative outcomes when undergoing procedures for revascularization. Even though there are well-established evidence-based therapies for treating acute coronary syndrome (ACS), guidelines and aggressive therapies are more likely to be applied in men. One of the most important factors in predicting survival and limiting myocardial damage in ACS is the time to revascularization. Due to delays in diagnosis and a perceived reluctance to treat women as aggressively, outcomes are often negatively affected.

As a society, we must make a concerted effort to close the gender gap in cardiovascular care. As physicians and healthcare providers, we must ensure that we apply the same practice guidelines and evidence-based therapies in both sexes. Women and their friends and families must advocate for their healthcare needs. Women must become more engaged in their own heart health in

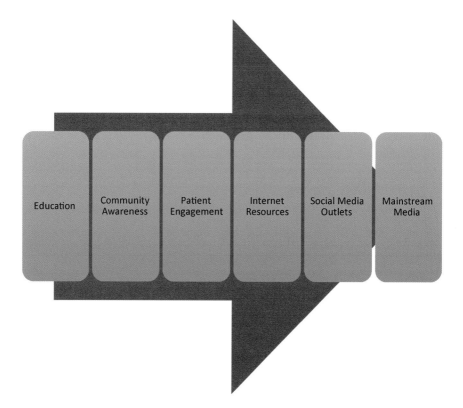

Figure 6.1 Strategies to close the gender gap in cardiovascular care for women.

order to effect change. The best way to effect change is to attack the problem of gender disparities in heart care from multiple fronts.

1. Education of Physicians and Healthcare Providers
2. Community Awareness Efforts
3. Patient Engagement & Individual Responsibility
4. Internet Resources
5. Social Media Outlets
6. Mainstream Media Efforts

Education of physicians and healthcare providers

Change must begin within the healthcare system. As physicians and healthcare providers we must recognize that the gender gap exists and then begin to educate ourselves on ways in which we can improve care for all women. Physicians are now busier than ever, seeing more patients in less time. Patients are living longer with chronic disease and a primary care visit can become increasingly complex. It can be difficult to tease out subtle symptoms and risk profiles in women that may suggest heart disease and indicate a need for further testing. However, we must begin to proactively screen our female patients on a regular basis.

So much of the successful doctor–patient relationship in medicine is dependent upon effective communication. Even with the added time pressures and the increased patient load, we must ensure that we take the time to actively engage with our female patients. Just as educators must understand the learning style of their students, physicians and healthcare providers we must do a better job understanding how each of their patients are best served during an office visits. Some patients prefer a more interactive and participatory style of encounter while others prefer a more dictatorial form of healthcare interaction. There is a large body of evidence in the literature that has examined the ways in which doctors and patients interact — many of these findings surprisingly indicate gender-specific differences.

Many women may be hesitant to discuss symptoms with their doctor and sometimes it takes several visits to get to know a patient well enough that she will begin to relax and open up during a visit. Data also supports the fact that there are differences in the ways in which female patients interact with male versus female doctors.[1]

---

[1] Beach, M. C. and Roter, D. L. (2000). Interpersonal Expectations in the Patient-physician Relationship. *J Gen Intern Med*, Volume 15(11), 825–827.

According to a study from the *New England Journal of Medicine*, female physicians are more likely to focus on preventative medicine and screening when compared with male colleagues.[2] More importantly, female physicians were found to be more likely to communicate in a way that involved the patient during the office visit — more of a participatory "two-way street" interaction.[3] Other studies have also demonstrated that female physicians are more likely to talk about lifestyle and habit modifications with patients in order to help prevent disease later in life.[4,5] Gender-specific patient characteristics also play a role in the doctor–patient interaction. Women tend to want to spend more time in the office visit and prefer to communicate more history and symptom information (once comfortable with their providers).[6] Female patients also seem to value more time spent by physicians explaining clinical situations than do male patients.[7] There is great power in better understanding how patients best engage. We must spend the time necessary to determine the best style for each patient — through engagement we are more likely to collect more relevant data and identify the at-risk female patient.

Beyond the doctor–patient interaction, much can be accomplished through physician education. By their very nature, healthcare

---

[2] Lurie, N., Slater, J., McGovern, P. *et al.* (1993). Preventive care for women: does the sex of the physician matter? *New Eng J Med*, Volume 329, 478–482.

[3] Cooper-Patrick, L., Gallo, J. J., Gonzales, J. J. *et al.* (1999). Race, gender, and partnership in the patient-physician relationship. *JAMA*, Volume 282, 583–589.

[4] Roter, D., Lipkin, M. and Korsgaard, A. (1991). Sex differences in patients' and physician's communication during primary care medical visits. *Med Care*, Volume 29, 1083–1093.

[5] Elderkin-Thompson, V. and Waitzkin, H. (1999). Differences in clinical communication by gender. *J Gen Intern Med*, Volume 14, 112–121.

[6] Wallen, J., Waitzkin, H. and Stoeckle J. (1979). Physician stereotypes about female health and illness: a study of patients' sex and the informative process during medical interviews. *Women Health*, Volume 4, 135–146.

[7] Hall, J. and Roter, D. (1988). Meta-analysis of correlates of provider behavior in medical encounters. *Med Care*, Volume 26, 651–659.

providers are scientists and respond well to data presented to them in order to effect changes in practice.[8] However, the way in which physician behavior is changed in response to evidence is not uniform and remains a complex issue. An important first step is to make sure that as a healthcare community, physicians and other providers are better educated about the gender disparities in cardiovascular care. There are many opportunities for continuing medical education at all levels — national meetings, continuing medical education (CME) conferences and local and regional medical society meetings are wonderful platforms for the discussion of women and heart disease. While there are some programs in place to address gender disparities in cardiac care, there is simply a paucity of large-scale emphasis. Even more important is the fact that many of the most common educational interventions that are made in practice today are relatively ineffective. Data from multiple analyses has shown that traditional CME programs with didactic and printed materials are ineffective unless these activities are combined with follow-up, clinical reminders and chart audits.[9] Adherence to guidelines significantly improves when traditional CME activities are combined with practice-specific follow-up activities that demonstrate change in physician behavior.

The best answer may be to create specific courses of study on women and heart disease and then help physicians develop chart reminder systems within their own electronic medical record systems. In addition, simple screening questionnaires have been developed by several organizations and these can be placed in the waiting room for female patients to complete while waiting for their appointments. Many of these screening questionnaires are based on a point system and can prompt the clinician to delve

[8] Smith, W. R. (2000). Evidence for the effectiveness of techniques to change physician behavior. *Chest*, Volume 118, 8S–17S.

[9] Bloom, B. S. (2005). Effects of continuing medical education on improving physician clinical care and patient health: A review of systematic reviews. *International Journal of Technology Assessment in Health Care*, Volume 21, 380–385.

deeper into a cardiac-specific discussion during the office encounter. Some institutions such as the Mayo Clinic have developed a gender-specific Women's Heart Clinic in order to serve the needs of female patients better.

No matter what approach we use, it is essential that all healthcare providers become more aware of the cardiovascular risks and the diagnostic challenges we face when treating women. We must work to assure that we educate ourselves, our colleagues and our patients about heart disease and its risk factors in order to effect change.

Community awareness efforts

Another critical component in closing the gender gap in cardiac care is better community education. We must not only ensure that physicians and other healthcare providers are aware of the disease prevalence in women; we must also make sure that those in our communities are aware of their own risk (and the risk of their family and friends). Campaigns such as the American Heart Association's Go Red For Women have been widely successful. Each year in February, a particular Friday is set aside as Wear Red Day. This event, and others like it, raise awareness and increase exposure to communities all over the country. Go Red events such as galas, dinners and fashion shows are able to raise funds for promoting women's health initiatives. The program encourages women of all ages to understand better and manage their risk for cardiovascular disease. These community-based awareness programs appear to be working but there is much more to be done. In a study published in 2012, researchers reported a significant increase in cardiovascular disease awareness among women between 1997 and 2012 — in fact, the rate of awareness nearly doubled from 30% to 56%.[10] However, in the same study, there were large gaps in awareness seen between different racial/ethnic groups.

---

[10]American Heart Association (2013). Fifteen-year trends in awareness of heart disease in women. *Circulation*, 10.1161/CIR.0b013e318287cf2f.

Other public forums for education such as women's social groups, business clubs, churches and fitness groups are also effective ways to improve women's knowledge of heart disease and its risk factors. Through improving awareness and through helping women in communities recognize risk we are able to assist them in making effective lifestyle changes to reduce risk of disease. Most importantly, community-based efforts spur conversation among women concerning heart disease. Hopefully these conversations will result in more detailed conversation with healthcare providers and ultimately reduce cardiovascular deaths in women.

Patient engagement and individual responsibility

As with most things in medicine, patient engagement is critical to success. As healthcare providers we must strive to assist our patients in making changes. However, we cannot do this alone. We must work together with our patients — help them identify their own risk and then assist each person in formulating an individualized plan for change. Patients must also accept individual responsibility for lifestyle modifications to reduce risk such as weight loss, diet, exercise and smoking cessation. A review of the literature demonstrates that the most effective way to effect change is to involve the patient in the treatment decision-making process and develop a partnership.[11] Both patient and doctor play a role and are held accountable for particular action items. No intervention will be successful without patient

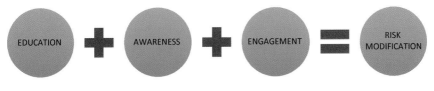

Figure 6.2   Process of patient engagement.

---

[11] Ong, L. M. L., de Haes, J. C. J. M., Hoos, A. M. *et al.* (1995). Doctor-patient communication: a review of the literature. *Soc Sci Med*, Volume 40, 903–918.

commitment. For example, in smoking cessation, regular follow-up is critical and making regular support mechanisms readily available to patients has been shown to increase both short term and long-term compliance rates.[12] Effective communication between physician and patient will create a sense of shared goals and will help to empower each woman to take charge of her own cardiovascular health.

Internet resources

In today's society nearly 60% of all adults have a smartphone or other mobile device. Most homes have at least one home computer and many are able to connect to the internet on a regular basis. The internet is widely available and offers access to vast amounts of information. Although quality control may be an issue with some websites — there are sites with valuable and reliable information. Many advocacy groups have taken advantage of this reach and have developed comprehensive websites targeted at women and heart disease. WomenHeart.org and GoRedForWomen.org are examples of quality internet resources. Laypeople can easily go to these sites for information and statistics surrounding heart disease in women. Moreover, when a healthcare professional is counseling a patient about heart disease and prevention these can be recommended reading for once the patient has left the office. Education experts have demonstrated that most people learn best and retain information most readily when they are exposed to concepts from multiple sources — in the case of heart disease and women these sources may include verbal doctor–patient interactions within the exam room, printed materials on heart disease and prevention and websites devoted to women's heart health. Patients who receive reinforcement and multiple points of contact are more likely to be successful in lifestyle and risk factor modifications. The internet is

---

[12] Ockene, J. K. (1987). Physician-delivered interventions for smoking cessation. Strategies for increasing effectiveness. *Preventive Medicine*, Volume 16, 723–737.

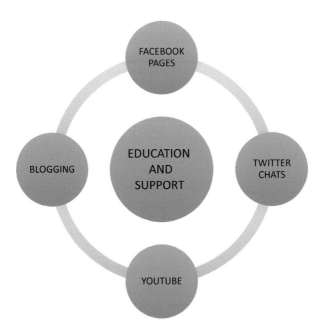

Figure 6.3 Social media resources.

another potential resource for both doctor and patient as they engage in care together.

In battling heart disease in women we must use every tool available to increase awareness and effect change.

Social media outlets

As mentioned previously, we are now a digital society. Many of us are active on social media networking sites such as Facebook and Twitter. These social media outlets can be powerful tools for change. Each of these outlets has their own following but all of them can be utilized effectively in medicine to disseminate information, engage patients, educate the public as well as create support groups. Currently, Facebook is the second most visited website in the world behind Google. Facebook can be a wonderful tool to educate patients and increase awareness about heart disease in women. For instance, a Facebook "Women's Heart Health Group Page" can be created and used as a platform to disseminate statistics about women and heart disease — ultimately resulting in improved community awareness. Twitter is a unique social media outlet that requires communication in 140 character messages. Twitter is valuable in that it can be used to create a buzz about an event (such as Go Red for Women) or it can draw attention to new developments in heart health that may appear on the news or in the press. Moreover, Twitter is an excellent venue to create virtual support groups. By identifying a particular conversation with a hashtag (#), a twitter chat can occur. Anyone who wants to join the chat simply searches for the tweets with the identified hashtag. For example, women who are working to stop smoking or reduce their risk for heart disease can join a chat that is identified as #womenshearthealth. These chats can be moderated by healthcare professionals and can serve as an effective means for encouraging lifestyle changes.

Mainstream media efforts

While social media and the internet are becoming more commonplace, the mainstream media remains a powerful tool for education and promoting community awareness of heart disease. The television media has improved their coverage of women's heart health issues in recent years. Most morning news shows feature stories on women and heart disease during the Go Red for Women campaigns. These stories are important to increase community awareness and often can spur conversation among viewers. However, the mainstream media can do much more. As healthcare providers it is essential that we actively interact with media personalities in order to promote women's heart health through interviews, promotional segments and charity events. Most local media professionals are always looking for stories that can directly impact the health of their viewers — stories on women and heart disease can have large and lasting effects.

Although we have made great strides in improving cardiovascular care for women in the last decade, gender disparities remain. As healthcare providers we must work tirelessly to improve community awareness of the risk of heart disease in women. We must educate and engage our patients and their families in order to effect real change. Women with heart disease continue to be undertreated and underserved. There is no one simple answer that will forever close this regrettable gap in care. However, we now have multiple resources that we must utilize to promote the identification and subsequent aggressive evidence-based treatment of both men *and* women with heart disease.

Chapter Seven

The Role of the OB/GYN in Improving Women's Cardiovascular Health

Traditionally, women have focused more on their gynecological health and screening rather than on cardiovascular risk. Most women, for instance, are far more concerned about developing breast cancer than having a heart attack or stroke. Yet, as we have discovered over the last decade, heart disease kills more women than all types of cancer combined. Breast cancer screening and awareness is much more prevalent among young women, but heart disease awareness is not. Because of the way in which women have increasingly actively adopted screening for breast and uterine/cervical cancer, many female patients faithfully see their gynecologist on an annual basis. Unfortunately, the number of women who regularly see a family physician or general internist *in addition to* the gynecologist is much smaller.

Yet these routine visits with the gynecologist do present an excellent opportunity for patient engagement, education and screening for heart disease. OB/GYN physicians are well trained and expert in all areas of gender-specific gynecologic disease, breast disease and other issues of women's health. However, when they are also faced with providing primary care services for their patients, they are often overwhelmed. Primary care is a specialty all to its own and those who train for the delivery of primary care spend countless hours in outpatient clinics and ambulatory care centers. In contrast, the OB/GYN physicians are trained as surgeons, who provide highly skilled surgical intervention for women with gynecological and obstetrical needs. Although they do have training in a clinical setting during residency, the bulk of their time is spent in the operating room. Most of their clinic-based work is focused on pre-operative and post-operative exams, pregnancy follow-up, and routine yearly gynecological exams. Nonetheless, many of these providers are faced with addressing primary care issues such as hypertension, depression, obesity and diabetes. They must rely on contacts with colleagues and referrals to specialists in order to ensure that their patients get the care they need. While many OB/GYN physicians do in fact counsel patients to obtain other primary care physicians for their general medicine needs, many of the patients simply refuse and assume that the OB/GYN will continue to treat all of their medical problems.

Primary care is defined as the practice of medicine that is focused on health promotion, disease prevention, health maintenance and patient education. In addition, primary care providers must also provide evaluation, diagnosis and treatment of acute medical problems. Ideally, the primary care provider is able to follow the patient over time and develop a long-standing relationship that allows for counseling, education and engagement. Many specialties are well prepared to delivery this type of care including Family Medicine, Internal Medicine and Pediatrics. However, many women choose to see only one provider and often that provider is the OB/GYN. Although this is less than ideal, it may represent an excellent opportunity to impact women's cardiovascular health. OB/GYN physicians tend to be passionate about the care of their patients and very willing to advocate for them.

How can the OB/GYN physician possibly meet the primary care needs of their patients?

The OB/GYN physician develops long-standing relationships with most of his or her patients due to the regularity of visits for annual screening and women's health maintenance. The relationship between women's health providers tends to have lifelong continuity of care. Continuity of care has been shown to be essential in patient engagement and providing positive outcomes.[1] In addition, women who have had children develop a special bond through the process of pregnancy and delivery with their OB/GYN physician. In many cases women with multiple children have had the same provider provide prenatal, pre-partum and post-partum care. This relationship results in a very high level of trust. When a female trusts another human being with the delivery of her child, a special bond is formed. For this reason, many women only trust their OB/GYN to provide care and are more apt to listen to them and comply with their recommendations.

When an OB/GYN is asked to provide primary care, they must assume a great responsibility. They must be willing to learn and educate others in their office about primary care issues. A key factor for successful primary care in a busy OBY/GYN office is the utilization of physician extenders such as nurse practitioners (NPs) and physician assistants (PAs). These practitioners tend to have more time to spend with each patient (which is a must when providing primary care visits). Extenders such as these are also trained in primary care as they receive their certifications and this allows them to be more prepared to screen and treat common medical problems. Most NPs and PAs are excellent communicators and enjoy spending time getting to know the patients on a personal level. The bond that is formed can be incredibly impactful on a provider's ability to engage with a

---

[1]Van Walraven, C., Oake, N., Jennings, A. *et al.* (2010). The association between continuity care and outcomes: a systematic and critical review. *J Eval Clin Pract*, Volume 16(5), 947–956.

patient and effect changes in lifestyle, diet and exercise — all of which are key components to the delivery of primary care.

Another critical element to the delivery of primary care in the OB/GYN office is the development of a strong referral network. Specialists such as endocrinologists, cardiologists, nephrologists and others can be essential in making sure that patients with specific medical problems get the care that they need. For instance, an OB/GYN may be perfectly capable of diagnosing type 2 diabetes in the office but certainly does not have the training or expertise to manage and adjust medication or insulin based on weekly blood sugar reports. In these cases, a referral to an endocrinologist may allow the patient to get optimal care and have more positive long-term outcomes. Coordination of care is paramount and communication amongst providers is essential for success — just as in any primary care setting.

How can the OB/GYN physician screen for heart disease?

As exclusive providers of healthcare for women, the OB/GYN physician is in a unique position to impact care and effect change in women's cardiovascular health. Women will make contact with the OB/GYN at least annually and this provides an excellent opportunity to screen for heart disease. In addition, when OB/GYN providers are educating patients about breast cancer screenings and the importance of self-exams at the annual visit they can also discuss heart disease risk factors and screening tests. As a whole, OB/GYN physicians are great educators and patient motivators — so much of prevention in gynecological disease requires patient engagement and patient education as to the risk and prevention of disease. For example, breast self-exams have been shown to be incredibly effective at detecting breast cancers in early stages — leading to better treatment options and more favorable long-term outcomes. In the case of screening for heart disease or its risk factors, simple questions can prompt further investigation and referral to a cardiologist for more advanced treatment and testing. Without this vital contact point with the OB/GYN provider, many women will go unnoticed and undiagnosed until they present with a potentially life-threatening cardiac event later in life.

But, as with most physicians, OB/GYN providers are overwhelmed with an increasing volume of patients and busy clinical schedules. How can these providers add additional responsibilities, such as screening for heart disease, into a routine clinic visit? One simple solution is to provide a "Risk Questionnaire" to patients as they sign in for their appointments in the waiting area. Data from previous studies have shown that self-administered cardiovascular screening tests are quite effective and reduce healthcare costs.[2] While patients wait for their turn in the exam room they can fill out a simple set of questions to evaluate their risk for heart disease. When the patient reaches the exam room, the nurse can review the questionnaire as part of the routine intake and alert the physician, NP or PA to a patient that provides worrisome answers on the screening tool. These patients are then identified to the providers as someone who will need more extensive screening and questioning during the office encounter. The American Heart Association has many useful tools for quick screening. These can be reproduced and placed in the office for use by patients. Many provide a quick score that predicts risk for future cardiovascular events. Obviously, those with low-risk scores can be simply counseled about the fact that women are at risk for disease and educated as to how to continue to remain low risk. Those with intermediate or high-risk scores can be actively treated and referred to other specialists for further testing and intervention.

How can the OB/GYN physician make a difference in cardiovascular death rates in women?

Engagement is key. Women tend to bond with their OB/GYN and trust them deeply. The OB/GYN thus has the opportunity to educate and engage the female patient in a way that may produce

---

[2]Cameron, J. D., Jennings, G. L., Kay, S. *et al.* (1997). A self-adminsitered questionnaire for detection of unrecognised coronary heart disease. *Aust N Z J Publica Health*, Volume 21(5), 545–547.

more positive cardiovascular outcomes. In addition, many women see the same OB/GYN for *life*. That means that a physician can engage with a young woman in her early 20s and follow her throughout her life. These physicians have the strength of long-term follow-up and an incredible continuity of care. Recent data has demonstrated that continuity of care in the treatment of diseases such as hypertension in younger patients may have a significant impact on cardiovascular events that occur later in life.[3] In this one particular study the trajectory of patient's blood pressure predicted the presence of heart disease later in life. Ultimately it argues for earlier screening and treatment of risk factors such as hypertension. This hypertension study is just one example where early intervention can make an enormous preventative difference. Given that OB/GYN physicians see women at early stages of adulthood, they have the opportunity to make a great impact. Additionally, hypertension during pregnancy has been shown to predict increase risk for stroke in women. Treatment guidelines from the American Heart Association warn of pregnancy-related hypertension and encourage timely treatment in order to decrease strokes in women later in life.[4] Clearly, OB/GYN providers may be able to play a critical role in the prevention of heart disease in women.

How can cardiologists help OB/GYN colleagues succeed in preventing heart disease?

One of the most important things that cardiologists, as non-OB/GYN providers, can do is to support and educate their colleagues. Events such as roundtable discussions and educational symposia

---

[3] Alllen, N. B., Siddique, J., Wilkins, J. T. *et al.* (2014). Blood pressure trajectories in early adulthood and subclinical artherosclerosis in middle age. *JAMA*, Volume 311(5), 490–497.

[4] AHA/ASA Guidelines (2014). A statement for healthcare professionals from the American Heart Association/American Stroke Association. 01.str.0000442009. 06663.48.

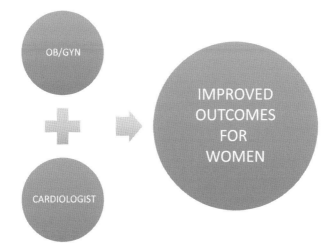

Figure 7.1   Cooperation of OB/GYN and cardiology providers.

directed specifically at OB/GYN physicians and extenders are critical to helping them feel comfortable with the diagnosis and screening of heart disease and its risk factors. Making sure that these providers understand the risk factors for heart disease, typical and atypical presentations of disease and (most importantly) when to *refer* patients is paramount in supporting them as they work to identify at-risk women. Although typical referral patterns in the past have not been established between OB/GYN providers and cardiologists (except in rare instances of peri-partum cardiomyopathies and other pregnancy-related cardiac complications), cardiologists must make it easy for their colleagues to refer and discuss patients with them. As specialists (as well as other primary care doctors), cardiologists must be easily reachable and readily available to provide help and support when the OB/GYN requests. Through cooperation amongst different specialties, we may be able to improve outcomes for women with heart disease.

Women continue to die from heart disease at alarming rates. The status quo is not working and more women continue to fall through the cracks. In order to reduce disease burden and improve outcomes for females, we must become innovative and find new ways to reach the at-risk women across the world. Engaging the OB/GYN in screening and diagnosing women with heart disease may be an important strategy. As providers of care to women all over the world, these specialists provide a unique opportunity to educate, engage and effect change in female patients. Ultimately, no specialty can handle the burden of heart disease alone — we must all work together to improve mortality and ensure that women are no longer undertreated and underserved.

Chapter Eight

Taking Control: Battling Obesity through Exercise

It is imperative that women engage with the prevention of heart disease. One of the most important lifestyle changes that women can make is the initiation and continuation of an active lifestyle. Our society has become more sedentary over the last 20 years and overall health status has suffered. In general, obesity is thought to contribute to the development of heart disease through the production of an increasing number of individuals with hypertension, diabetes and hyperlipidemia. In fact, a study published in the *New England Journal of Medicine* in 1990 found that, in women, obesity was a strong predictor of coronary artery disease.[1] In the study, women were divided into quartiles based on their weight and size, and researchers found that in women in the highest quartile for weight, there was a three-fold increase in fatal myocardial infarction and cardiovascular death, as compared to leaner women.[1]

Women who are obese may be more likely to develop metabolic syndrome, which has been associated with an increased risk of heart disease and stroke. According to the National Heart,

---

[1] Mason, J., Colditz, G. A., Stampfer, M. J. *et al.* (1990). A Prospective study of obesity and risk of coronary heart disease in women. *NEJM*, Volume 322, 882–889.

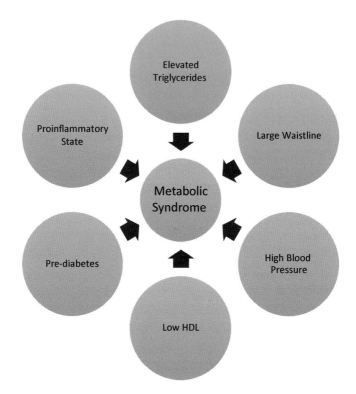

Figure 8.1   The metabolic syndrome and heart disease.

Lung and Blood Institute, metabolic syndrome is defined as having at least three of the following risk factors: (1) large waistline (apple shape), (2) elevated triglycerides, (3) low HDL (high-density lipoprotein), (4) high blood pressure, (4) elevated fasting blood sugar or pre-diabetes, (5) proinflammatory state and (6) prothrombotic state.[2] Elevated fasting blood sugar is an important component of metabolic syndrome and is associated with

[2]Grundy, S. M., Bryan Brewer, H. Jr., Cleeman, J. I. *et al.* (2004). Definition of metabolic syndrome report of the National Heart, Lung and Blood Institute/ American Heart Association conference on scientific issues related to definition. *NHLBI/AHA Conference Proceedings*, Volume 109, 433–438.

insulin resistance, which has been demonstrated to be a potent contributor to the development of heart disease.

Metabolic syndrome is becoming more commonplace among women as obesity levels rise. In fact, it is estimated that metabolic syndrome may eventually overtake smoking as a leading risk factor for heart disease, both in the US and abroad. It is critical that women recognize the symptoms of metabolic syndrome and intervene early to reduce their risk of heart disease and stroke. The individual components, as mentioned above, have been indentified as significant contributors to the development of heart disease. Abdominal obesity is most strongly associated with metabolic syndrome and is manifested as increase in waistline circumference. Lipid abnormalities are characterized by a very atherogenic combination of low HDL, high triglycerides and increased amounts of low-density lipoprotein particles.[2] Hypertension has long been associated with vascular damage and stiffness of the arteries. Insulin resistance strongly correlates to cardiovascular disease risk and results in elevated serum glucose levels — which are strongly associated with the development of cardiovascular disease. Inflammation is a major contributor to heart disease and can be measured by elevations of C-reactive protein (CRP). Obesity has been shown to promote the release of inflammatory cytokines, which, in turn, result in higher levels of CRP.[3] There is an increasing body of evidence that suggests that elevated CRP levels are associated with higher risk for heart disease.[4] The final component, the prothrombotic state, occurs when there are higher levels of circulating clotting factors such as fibrinogen. Similar to CRP, these levels also rise with the elevation of cytokines in the bloodstream and may be interconnected. The elevation of clotting factors may contribute to the formation of plaques in the coronary

---

[3]Yudkin, J. S., Stehouwer, C. D. A., Emeis, J. J. *et al.* (1999). C-reactive protein in healthy subjects: associations with obesity, insulin resistance, and endothelial dysfunction. *Arterioscler Thromb Vasc Biol*, Volume 19, 972–978.

[4]Ridker, P. M. (2003). Clinical application of C-reactive protein for cardiovascular disease detection and prevention. *MD Circulation*, 107: 363–369.

arteries and promote the development of heart attacks in women with metabolic syndrome.[5]

Obesity is defined as a BMI of more than 30. BMI is calculated by taking the body weight in kilograms and dividing by the height in meters squared. This standard measure allows for standard comparison of multiple body types. Research has shown that BMI correlates quite well with an individual's body fat composition.[6] Interestingly, women tend to have more body fat at similar BMI levels as compared to men.[7] Older adults tend to also have more body fat at similar BMI levels when compared to younger people.

The Centers for Disease Control (CDC) in the US has defined standard cutoff points for BMI for the purpose of defining levels of obesity, and these are based on recommendations for the World Health Organization. It is important to remember that these BMI standards are applicable only in those over 18 years of age — in children a different interpretation is utilized. Standard tables from the World Health Organization for BMI definitions are displayed in Table 8.1.

BMI has been shown to have a direct correlation with mortality in both men and women. In a recent publication, Adams *et al.* demonstrated that when compared to patients with normal BMIs, those with a BMI over 25 (and those that attained that BMI earlier in life) were found to have higher all-cause mortality.[8] In fact, both weight

[5] Juhan-Vague, I., Thompson, S. G. and Jespersen, J. (1993). Involvement of the hemo-static system in the insulin resistance syndrome: a study of 1500 patients with angina pectoris. *Arterioscler Thromb*, Volume 13, 1865–1873.

[6] Mei, Z., Grummer-Strawn, L. M., Pietrobelli, A. *et al.* (2002). Validity of body mass index compared with other body-composition screening indexes for the assessment of body fatness in children and adolescents. *American Journal of Clinical Nutrition*, Volume 75(6), 7597–7985.

[7] Gallagher, D., Visser, M., Sepúlveda, D. *et al.* (1996). How useful is BMI for comparison of body fatness across age, sex and ethnic groups? *American Journal of Epidemiology*, Volume 143, 228–239.

[8] Adams, K. F., Leitzmann, M. F., Ballard-Barbash, R. *et al.* (2014). Body mass and weight change in adults in relation to mortality risk. *Am J Epidemiol*, Volume 179(2), 135–144.

Table 8.1   The international classification of adult underweight, overweight and obesity according to BMI.

Classification	BMI (kg/m2)	
	Principal cutoff points	Additional cutoff points
Underweight	**<18.50**	**<18.50**
Severe thinness	<16.00	<16.00
Moderate thinness	16.00–16.99	16.00–16.99
Mild thinness	17.00–18.49	17.00–18.49
Normal range	**18.50–24.99**	**18.50–22.99**
		23.050–24.99
Overweight	**≥25.00**	**≥25.00**
Pre-obese	25.00–29.99	25.00–27.49
		27.50–29.99
Obese	**≥30.00**	**≥30.00**
Obese class I	30.00–34.99	30.00–32.49
		32.50–34.99
Obese class II	35.00–39.99	35.00–37.49
		37.50–39.99
Obese class III	≥40.00	≥40.00

Source: Adapted from WHO, 1995, WHO, 2000, and WHO, 2004.

gain and BMI at all ages were directly related to all-cause mortality. It is clear that obesity is a key component in the development of chronic disease. In women, obesity may be an even more significant risk factor for the development of coronary artery disease, particularly given the relationship of obesity to metabolic syndrome.

Today, obesity and obesity-related illness is a 190 billion dollar healthcare expense in the US alone and accounts for nearly 21% of all healthcare expenditures.[9] Obesity is clearly related to the development of diabetes, heart disease, hypertension and other

---

[9] Cawley, J. and Meyerhoefer, C. (2012). The medical care costs of obesity: an instrumental variables approach. *Journal of Health Economics*, Volume 31(1), 219–230.

chronic illnesses. Interestingly, obesity affects women differently than men. As mentioned previously, women tend to have higher body fat composition at similar BMI levels and thus increased risk for heart disease at lower levels of BMI. Obesity in women may produce increased risk through the promotion of insulin resistance. In fact, in a study of nearly 37,000 women, those with a BMI greater than 35 were significantly more likely to have coronary artery disease as well as hypertension.[10] Other studies have demonstrated that obesity is an independent risk factor for heart disease in women.[11] Abdominal fat deposition and the "apple shape" has been shown to be a very powerful predictor of heart disease in women — in a study of nearly 7,000 women from 52 countries this body type was found to be a more powerful predictor of myocardial infarction or heart attack than BMI alone.[12] Data from the Nurses' Health Study involving over 44,000 women demonstrated a relative risk for death from heart disease of nearly 3.5 in those with a waist circumference of more than 44 cm.[13] The evidence for the negative effects of obesity in women and cardiovascular mortality is powerful and argues for early intervention. In addition, it is clear that obesity affects both men and women in different ways and may provide a more significant contribution of risk in female patients.

Obesity is clearly directly related to physical inactivity and those who are more physically active are less likely to be obese. A study in *Circulation* published in 2006, actually showed that both *obesity* and *physical inactivity* are independent predictors of

[10] Patterson, R. E., Frank, L. L., Kristal, A. R. *et al.* (2004). A comprehensive examination of health conditions associated with obesity in older adults. *Am J Prev Med*, Volume 27, 385–390.

[11] Weiss, A. M. (2009). Cardiovascular disease in women. *Prim Care*, Volume 36, 73–102.

[12] Anand, S. S., Islam, S., Rosengren, A. *et al.* (2008). Risk factors for myocardial infarction in women and men: in- sights form the INTERHEART study. *Eur Heart J*, Volume 29, 932–940.

[13] Carey, V. J., Walters, E. E., Colditz, G. A. *et al.* (1997). Body fat distribution and risk of non-insulin-dependent dia- betes mellitus in women, Nurses' Health Study. *Am J Epidemiol*, Volume 145, 614–619.

the development of heart disease.[14] This finding further emphasizes not only the importance of maintaining a healthy body weight, but also the importance of daily exercise, particularly in women.

Initial investigations that demonstrated a positive relationship between exercise and heart disease risk were performed in patient populations that were predominantly made up of male subjects. Subsequent investigations were done in the last ten years that focused solely on female patients. It is clear from numerous studies that active women experience less heart disease than those who are sedentary.[15] However, what is less clear is the exact nature of the type and duration of physical activity required in order to make a difference in cardiovascular outcomes. Many experts have advocated a rigorous exercise program while others have argued for a more moderate-to-low-intensity exercise routine.[16,17] We have now come to learn that even light-to-moderate physical activity confers a significantly lower risk of cardiovascular disease in women. In fact, research published in the *Journal of the American Medical Association* in 2001 demonstrated that even one hour of walking per week resulted in a lower cardiovascular mortality in a large group of female subjects.[18] From this investigation it was concluded that the time spent exercising or walking was far more important than the intensity or pace. *Any* activity seemed to confer benefit as compared to a more sedentary lifestyle. The CDC's recommendations of at least 150 minutes per week of

---

[14] Li, T. Y., Rana, J. S., Manson, J. E. *et al.* (2006). Obesity as compared with physical activity in predicting risk of coronary heart disease in women. *Circulation*, Volume 113, 499–506.

[15] Sesso, H. D. (1999). Physical activity and cardiovascular disease risk in women. *Am J Epidemiology*, Volume 150, 408–416.

[16] Lea and Febiger (1985). *Guidelines for Graded Exercise Testing and Exercise Prescription*, 3rd ed. New York: American College of Sports Medicine.

[17] Pate, R. R., Pratt, M., Blair, S. N. *et al.* (1995). Physical activity and public health: a recommendation from the Centers for Disease Control and Prevention and the American College of Sports Medicine. *JAMA*, Volume 273, 402–407.

[18] Lee, I. M., Rexrode, K. M., Cook, N. R. *et al.* (2001). Physical activity and coronary heart disease in women. *JAMA*, Volume 285, 1447–1454.

moderate-intensity exercise for adults are supported by these findings. The CDC goes on to remark that this 150 minutes broken up into easily manageable blocks of time — even as little as ten minutes at a time — will result in lower risk for cardiovascular disease.

What does this mean for women?

Most importantly, these findings suggest that we, as physicians, must encourage women to exercise on a daily basis. No matter what a particular individual's level of fitness is, they can benefit from light-to-moderate daily exercise. We now know that any activity confers improved survival when compared to a sedentary lifestyle. For female patients, this should serve as a call to action. As healthcare providers, we must empower women to accept responsibility and take control. One very effective way to take control is through lifestyle modification and exercise. Through education and support, we can help any female patient (or friend, mother, sister or child) to begin to transform their cardiovascular risk profile through exercise. It is important, however, that as we encourage women to engage in physical activity we help them do so in a safe and reasonable way.

Taking the first steps

It is essential that all healthcare providers include counseling about physical activity with their patients as part of routine office visits — irrespective of specialty. It is clear that the more a patient hears a message, the more likely they are to adopt a lifestyle change. We must educate patients about the benefits of exercise and also assess their particular level of fitness in order to assist them in their exercise plan. For some patients, evaluation with stress testing may be necessary. For others, it is as simple as a basic history and physical exam.

When embarking on a new exercise regimen, patients must have realistic expectations. It is important that women understand just how important exercise is to their overall health status and that *any* exercise at *any* level of exertion provides benefit. Each individual

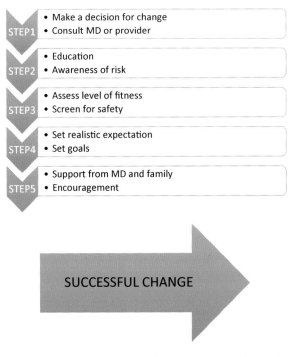

Figure 8.2 Beginning exercise: the process of making a change.

patient will have to determine exactly what type of plan will work best for them — for some, group activities are important while for others, walking at home or working out at a gym may be more beneficial. Personal training may be an option for some patients. Others may have orthopedic issues related to their weight and these patients benefit from water-based exercises such as water aerobics. However, the bottom line for all women is that exercise is an essential step in the prevention of obesity and ultimately cardiovascular disease.

As physicians, we must provide support and encouragement. It is important that we help them set reasonable weight loss and fitness goals and provide a framework and a plan for achieving these goals. We must help them celebrate successes and support them when they do not meet their goals. As mentioned previously, when doctors and patients are able to partner and work together to manage chronic disease, outcomes improve. Obesity is slowly destroying the health of American women. Unless we make major interventions *now*, it is estimated that by the year 2030 nearly 50% of all Americans will be considered obese — in some states obesity rates are predicted to be in excess of 60%.[19] Exercise and a change in lifestyle can be one of the most effective preventive tools for women to use to take charge and reduce their own risk for cardio-vascular events.

---

[19] Fiester, L. (2014). Trust for America's health examines states' obesity rates and related costs. *RFJ*, available online at: http://www.rwjf.org/en/research-publications/find-rwjf-research/2014/01/trust-for-america-s-health-examines-states--obesity-rates-and-re.html. Accessed 29 April 2014.

Chapter Nine

Taking Control: Battling Obesity through Dietary Change and Stress Management

As we have discussed in previous chapters, obesity is epidemic in the US and abroad. Obesity and obesity-related illness account for nearly 190 billion dollars of annual healthcare expenditure in the US alone. Obese women are at particular risk for cardiovascular disease and must do more to moderate their risk. Engagement is critical. In the last chapter, we discussed the importance of lifestyle modification — particularly exercise — in reducing risk.

However, exercise is just one, albeit important, piece of the puzzle. Obesity is clearly related to caloric intake, lifelong habits and dietary choices. Women must accept individual responsibility for their own cardiovascular health and partner with their healthcare providers in order to effect change. Managing weight with diet and exercise is not an easy task and requires dedication and hard work. Dietary changes often require support of family and friends and it is typically necessary for patients to ask family to make changes with them as they embark upon a weight loss journey. More importantly, patients must change habits in order to *maintain* weight loss. Numerous studies on diet and weight loss have indicated that long-term maintenance of weight loss can be quite challenging and results have been less than ideal.[1,2] In a meta-analysis of obese individuals who participated in structured weight loss programming, most only maintained approximately 23% of their total weight loss at year five.[3] Data from the National Weight Control Registry has been analyzed over the years and has helped physicians and nutritionists to identify characteristics that may predict those that are more likely to be unsuccessful with maintenance of weight loss.[4] The following characteristics are associated with those that are more likely to be successful with weight loss over the long term when employing a strategy of diet modification[5]:

(1) Concomitant participation in high levels of physical activity
(2) Consuming a diet that is low in calories and fat
(3) Never skipping breakfast
(4) Regular self monitoring of weight
(5) Maintaining a constant eating pattern — no binging
(6) Catching "slips" early

Interestingly, studies from this same registry indicated that weight loss after any significant "medical event" seemed to help to facilitate long-term weight control.[6] When patients were asked, nearly 83% of those in the registry reported a significant event as the trigger for their engagement in dietary plans for weight loss.

---

[1]Anderson, T., Backer, O. G., Stockholm, K. H. *et al.* (1984). Randomized trial of diet and gastroplasty with diet alone in morbid obesity. *N Engl J Med*, Volume 310, 352–356.
[2]Brownell, K. D. and Jeffrey, R. W. (1987). Improving long-term weight loss: pushing the limits of treatment. *Behav Ther*, Volume 18, 353–374.
[3]Anderson, J. W., Konz, E. C., Frederich, R. C. *et al.* (2001). Long-term weight-loss maintenance: a meta-analysis of US studies. *Am J Clin Nutr*, November, Volume 74(5), 579–584.
[4]McGuire, M. T., Wing, R. R., Klem, M. L. *et al.* (1999). What predicts weight regain in a group of successful weight losers? *J Consult Clin Psychol*, Volume 67, 177–185.
[5]Wing, R. R. and Phelan, S. (2005). Long-term weight loss maintenance. *Am J Clin Nutr*, July, 82(1), 222S–225S.
[6]Gorin, A., Phelan, S., Hill, J. A. *et al.* (2004). Medical triggers are associated with better long-term weight maintenance. *Prev Med*, Volume 39, 612–616.

Triggering events were found to be medical in 23%, reaching an all-time-high weight in 21% and seeing a picture or reflection of themselves in 12%.[6] Medical triggers for weight loss were associated with greater total weight loss and better weight maintenance over the long term. Many of these medically motivated patients in the registry were those who had suffered a cardiac event and were told to "lose weight" by their cardiologist or internist after the acute phase of the illness was survived. This data suggests that the time following a medical trigger may be a very opportune time for intervention with patients to promote more successful long-term weight loss. Physicians and other healthcare providers should utilize this time to actively influence patients and families to initiate lifestyle changes and improve outcomes. As we have seen in previous chapters, obesity seems to be a particularly significant modifiable risk factor in women and the reduction of BMI may result in lower rates of cardiovascular disease and acute cardiac events.

Just as with daily exercise and physical activity, it is essential to empower women with the knowledge they need to be successful. We must engage and motivate patients so that they are willing to actively participate in their care and in both the primary and (if necessary) secondary prevention of cardiovascular disease.

Which diet is right? Offering guidance for improved cardiovascular outcomes

There are many choices when it comes to dietary regimens aimed at improving cardiovascular health and reducing body weight. Many of these diets have been well studied and outcomes are published in peer-reviewed medical journals. The American Heart Association has advocated a low fat diet with only 30% of calories from fat — however, this often results in high degrees of carbohydrate intake which can lead to obesity, insulin resistance and weight gain.[7]

---

[7] Krauss, R. M., Eckel, R. H., Howard, B. *et al.* (2000). AHA dietary guidelines, revision 2000: A statement for healthcare professionals from the Nutrition Committee of the American Heart Association. *Circulation*, Volume 102, 2296–2311.

There are several major dietary approaches that have been considered to be key in the prevention of cardiovascular disease. Each of these has been well studied in the medical literature and each has risks and benefits associated with them.

(1) Low carbohydrate diets: Carbohydrate restrictive diets such as the Atkins diet have been practiced for many years.[8] These diets rely upon carbohydrate restriction initially, followed by gradual reintroduction. In contrast to the American Heart Association (AHA) guidelines, diets such as the Atkins approach obtain nearly 70% of the daily calories from fat. When multiple studies involving low carbohydrate diets are reviewed, it is noted that HDL (high-density lipoprotein) cholesterol improves to higher levels while LDL (low-density lipoprotein) cholesterol and triglyceride levels are significantly reduced.[9] Over time, total weight loss is not appreciably different from other dietary strategies. Unfortunately most trials involved small patient numbers and did not involve lengthy follow-up times so any real impact on cardiovascular mortality is difficult to determine in any statistically significant way.

(2) Glycemic index diets: The glycemic index (GI) is a measure of blood glucose response to intake of a particular carbohydrate type and the higher the blood glucose response, the higher the GI assigned.[10] Studies have shown that diets with high values for glycemic index are associated with higher rates of obesity, diabetes and cardiovascular disease.[11] It appears that diets that consist of foods that rapidly raise the blood sugar level may actually increase levels of free fatty acids and play a role in the

---

[8] Atkins, R. C. (1998). *Dr. Atkins' New Diet Revolution*. New York: Avon Books.

[9] Bravata, D. M., Sander, L., Huang, J. *et al.* (2003). Efficacy and safety of low-carbohydrate diets: a systematic review. *JAMA*, Volume 289, 1837–1850.

[10] Jenkins, D. J. A., Thomas, D. M., Wolever, S. *et al.* (1981). Glycemic index of food: a physiological basis for carbohydrate exchange. *Am J Clin Nutr*, Volume 34, 362–366.

[11] Lefebvre, P. J. and Scheen, A. J. (1998). The postprandial state and risk of cardiovasular disease. *Diabet Med*, Volume 15, S63–S68.

induction of endothelial injury and the activation of coagulation through oxidative stress. Endothelial injury and hypercoagulability contribute to the process of plaque formation in the development of coronary artery disease.[11] Although many of these diets have been effective in promoting weight loss, there are no clinical trials that have shown that diets that promote a low GI are associated with a lower risk for cardiovascular disease.

(3) Low fat diets: Very low fat diets (VLFD) are defined as diets that include no more than 15% of total calories from fat (with an equal amount of saturated and polyunsaturated fats). Many vegetarian diets rely on the very low fat concept. There does appear to be some association between the VLFD and decreased cardiovascular risk.[12] This diet is often very restrictive and can be difficult for many patients to adhere to.

(4) Mediterranean diet: The Mediterranean diet has well-established evidence in the reduction of cardiovascular disease.[13] In addition, there are large databases that have demonstrated that adherence to the Mediterranean-style diet is associated with a significant reduction in obesity.[14] In general, the Mediterranean diet consists of olive oil as the principal fat, lots of fruits, vegetables, nuts and legumes, and the primary protein in the form of fish. Meat and dairy intake is minimized and daily moderate alcohol consumption in the form of red wine with meals is encouraged.[15] This type of diet has been associated with lower BMIs, lower fasting glucose levels, lower blood pressure and lower levels of circulating inflammatory markers such as

---

[12] Lichtenstein, A. H. and Van Horn, L. (1998). AHA science advisory: very low fat diets. *Circulation*, Volume 98, 935–939.

[13] Martinez-Gonzalez, M. A. and Sanchez-Villegas, A. (2004). The emerging role of Mediterranean diets in cardiovascular epidemiology: monounsaturated fats, olive oil, red wine or the whole pattern? *Eur J Epidemiol*, Volume 19, 9–13.

[14] Mendez, M. A., Popkin, B. M. and Jakszyn, P. (2006). Adherence to a Mediterranean diet is associated with reduced 3-year incidence of obesity. *J Nutr*, Volume 136, 2934–2938.

[15] Trichopoulou, A., Orfanos, P., Norat, T. *et al.* (2005). Modified Mediterranean diet and survival: EPIC-elderly prospective cohort study. *BMJ*, Volume 330, 991.

C-reactive protein (CRP). When elevated, all of these markers have been associated with higher risk of cardiovascular disease and death. Even in patients who have experienced a previous myocardial infarction, adoption of the Mediterranean-style diet has been associated with a significantly lower risk of cardiac death in these secondary prevention patients.[16]

Special dietary considerations in women

There have been numerous studies that have examined specific dietary changes in women and the impacts these changes have on cardiovascular disease incidence as well as cardiovascular-related deaths. Lessons learned from these studies that were conducted with only women subjects can provide important insights into how specific changes can make a difference in risk for disease.

For example, there has been much research done on the impact of dietary fats on heart disease. It has been proven that the intake of high quantities of trans fats is associated with higher risk for heart disease.[17] Trans fats are synthetic fats that can give food a pleasing texture and taste. They are rarely found naturally but are easily produced by industry and are also found in hydrogenated oils. Trans fats are widely utilized in the fast food industry due to the fact that they are easy to produce in a cost-effective and profitable way. In addition, many crackers, cookies, cakes and fried foods contain trans fats. The FDA is currently considering legislation to ban or severely limit the use of trans fats in the food supply, given the high association of trans fats with cardiovascular disease.[18]

---

[16]Trichopoulou, A., Bamia, C. and Trichopoulos, D. (2005). Mediterranean diet and survival among patients with coronary heart disease in Greece. *Arch Intern Med*, Volume 165, 929–935.

[17]Willett, W. C., Stampfer, M. J., Manson, J. E. *et al.* (1993). Intake of trans fatty acids and risk of coronary heart disease among women. *Lancet*, Volume 341, 581–585.

[18]FDA (2013). Tentative determination regarding partially hydrogenated oils. *Federal Register*, Volume 78(217), 67169–67175.

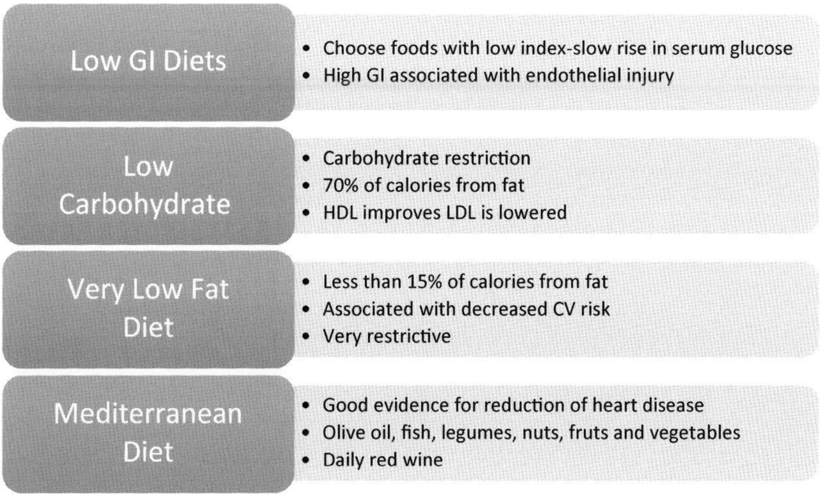

Figure 9.1 Common diet options and heart disease. CV = cardiovascular disease.

A study from the *New England Journal of Medicine* from 1997, evaluated the role of fat consumption in women and rates of heart disease.[19] In this investigation, the relationship between dietary intake of specific types of fats — trans saturated, monounsaturated and polyunsaturated and the risk of coronary artery disease was examined in women who were part of the Nurses' Health Study database. Involving over 80,000 women, the study found that each increase of 5% of energy intake from saturated fat resulted in a 17% increase in coronary artery disease risk. Moreover, the intake of polyunsaturated and monounsaturated fats did not result in a statistically significant increase in cardiovascular disease risk. Most importantly, total fat intake was not associated with increased heart disease risk *but* replacing saturated fats with poly- and monounsaturated fats resulted in a 53% reduction in cardiovascular disease risk.[17] The authors concluded that replacing saturated and trans saturated fats with mono- and polyunsaturated fats is more effective in preventing heart disease than simply reducing overall fat intake.

---

[19] Hu, F. B., Stampfer, M. J., Manson, J. E. *et al.* (1997). Dietary fat intake and the risk of coronary heart disease in women. *NEJM*, Volume 337, 1491–1499.

These data have real implications for women as they make dietary changes and work to take control of their own modifiable risks — learning to read food labels and select products that have more favorable fat compositions is critical to risk reduction.

As we have mentioned earlier in the chapter, the Mediterranean diet has been shown to decrease cardiovascular mortality in both men and women. A staple of the Mediterranean-style diet is the consumption of nuts and legumes. Now, in addition to looking at the types of fats that are consumed, there are also studies that have been conducted in women to evaluate the cardiovascular benefits of nuts. In a study from Harvard published in 1998, researchers evaluated the effects of frequent nut consumption on women and their cardiovascular health. What they found was a powerful reduction in both fatal coronary heart disease and non-fatal myocardial infarction.[20] In fact, women who consumed nuts more than five times a week had a 35% reduction in cardiovascular events as compared to those women who rarely ate nuts. Other studies such as the *Adventist Health Study*, also demonstrated a positive effect of nut consumption — nearly a 50% reduction in risk for cardiovascular disease.[21]

Data for dietary modification in the reduction of heart disease is compelling. While women cannot control their family history or genetic predisposition to disease, obesity- and diet-related risk are things that can be modified through engagement and dedication to change.

What is ultimately the right choice?

The right choice is ultimately the diet that brings success. Each individual must choose a diet and make a lifestyle change that they

---

[20] Hu, F. B., Stampfer, M. J., Manson, J. E. *et al.* (1998). Frequent nut consumption and risk of coronary heart disease in women: prospective cohort study. *BMJ*, Volume 317, 1341.

[21] Fraser, G. E., Sabate, J., Beeson, W. L. *et al.* (1992). A possible protective effect of nut consumption on risk of coronary heart disease. The Adventist Health Study. *Arch Intern Med*, Volume 152, 1416–1424.

are able to adhere to *and* enjoy. As healthcare providers, we must make recommendations and help our patients choose the plan that will give them the best chance of achieving their goals. Diets that focus solely on elimination have lower success rates than those that focus more on including multiple healthy food choices. Lifestyle changes, such as diets, require support. As physicians and providers of healthcare to women, we must work to provide a network of support for our patients. This can be accomplished through routine follow-ups as well as the creation of patient-based support groups within the practice.

Research indicates that social support systems — particularly family support — can make an enormous difference in the success of any weight loss plan.[22] As healthcare providers for women, it is essential that we involve families, including children and spouses, in any lifestyle modification plan. If we are able to involve and engage loved ones as well as the patient, we can facilitate changes in behavior that will assist in reducing cardiovascular death in women.

In addition to family support, there is a growing body of evidence that suggests that internet and online support for weight loss programs is equivalent to the effects of face-to-face support groups.[23] In fact, results from a study in 2004 show that a weight maintenance program based solely on internet interaction could sustain comparable long-term weight loss to those conducted in person or via telephone. The fact that alternative support opportunities exist allows us to provide even more options for our patients who wish to lose weight. The proliferation of online tools and the internet allows even those with limited access to transportation to take full advantage of the support systems that breed success.

---

[22] Marcouxa, B. C., Trenknerb, L. L. and Rosenstockc, I. M. (1990). Social networks and social support in weight loss. *Patient Education and Counseling*, Volume 15, 229–238.

[23] Harvey-Berino, J., Pintauro, S., Buzzell, P. *et al.* (2004). Effect of internet support on the long-term maintenance of weight loss. *Obesity Research*, Volume 12(2), 320–329.

What about stress and heart disease in women?

Stress has been identified as a significant risk factor for chronic disease for quite some time and has been associated with premature aging and increased risk for heart disease and stroke.[24, 25] There is clearly a link between the mind and the body and exogenous life stressors have a negative effect on our bodies. While not much is known about the precise mechanism by which this occurs, at the molecular level cellular damage is mediated by shortened telomeres.[26] Telomeres are caps on the end of chromosomes, which work to maintain chromosomal stability. It is postulated that shortened telomeres are associated with increased cellular damage and accelerated aging. Moreover, antioxidants have been found to protect against cellular damage via limiting the shortening of telomeres.[27]

We have discussed previously that women often find themselves under a great deal of stress. In one study, it was found that reported psychological stressors in a group of women was significantly associated with increased oxidative stress, shortened telomeres and reduced telomere function at the cellular level.[28] In addition, women with increased stress were found to have one decade of additional biological age (at the cellular level). These findings may help explain how stress can significantly impact women's risk for heart disease and stroke.

---

[24] McEwen, B. (1998). Seminars in medicine of the Beth Israel Deaconess Medical Center: Protective and damaging effects of stress mediators. *N Engl J Med*, Volume 338, 171–179.

[25] Segerstrom, S. and Miller, G. (2004). Psychological stress and the human immune system: a meta-analytic study of 30 years of inquiry. *Psychol Bull*, Volume 130(4), 601–630.

[26] Chan, S. R. and Blackburn, E. H. (2004). Telomeres and telomerase. *Philos Trans R Soc London B*, Volume 359(1441), 109–121.

[27] Irie, M., Asami, S., Ikeda, M. *et al.* (2003). Depressive state relates to female oxidative DNA damage via neutrophil activation. *Biochem Biophys Res Commun*, Volume 311, 1014–1018.

[28] Epel, E. S., Blackburn, E. H., Lin, J., *et al.* (2004). Accelerated telomere shortening in response to life stress. *PNAS*, Volume 101(49), 17312–17315.

There have been other studies that have shown a significant association between increased perceived stress and risk of cardiovascular death. Shift work has been long associated with increased rates of stress and serves as a good model for clinical investigation of the effects of long-term stress on survival.[29] A study published in *Circulation* in 1995 demonstrated an increased risk for cardiovascular disease in women with increased psychological stress due to shift work.[30]

Other syndromes such as Takotsubo's "broken heart syndrome" provide a clear link between stress in women and heart disease.[31] In this model, extreme emotional or physical stress in women results in apical ballooning of the heart and can mimic an acute myocardial infarction. It is clear that in women there is a direct link between stress and cardiovascular abnormalities. It is postulated that the emotional or physical stress results in an activation of the neurohormonal axis and causes a surge in catecholamines. The high levels of catecholamines have been thought to induce coronary vasospasm, microvascular vasospasm and even cellular injury to cardiac myocytes.[32,33] Luckily with Takotsubo's syndrome, the damage is reversible and most patients are able to return to normal life with a normal heart as long as they are able to control their response to stress adequately.

---

[29] Coffey, L. C., Skipper, J. K. and Jung, F. D. (1998). Nurses and shift work: effects on job performance and job-related stress. *J Adv Nursing*, Volume 13, 245–254.

[30] Kawachi, I. (1995). Prospective study of shift work and risk of coronary heart disease in women. *Circulation*, Volume 92, 3178–3182.

[31] Gianni, M., Dentali, F., Grandi A. M. *et al.* (2006). Apical ballooning syndrome or takotsubo cardiomyopathy: a systematic review. *Eur Heart J*, Volume 27(13), 1523–1529.

[32] Kurisu, S., Inoue, I., Kawagoe, T. *et al.* (2004). Time course of electrocardiographic changes in patients with tako-tsubo syndrome: comparison with acute myocardial infarction with minimal enzymatic release. *Circ J*, Volume 68, 77–81.

[33] Abe, Y., Kondo, M., Matsuoka, R. *et al.* (2003). Assessment of clinical features in transient left ventricular apical ballooning. *J Am Coll Cardiol*, Volume 41, 737–742.

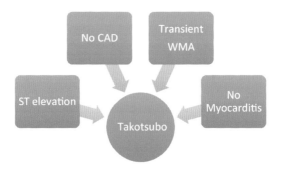

Figure 9.2   Diagnostic features of Takotsubo's "stress-induced" cardiomyopathy. WMA = wall motion abnormality.

Emotional and psychological stressors have been proven to increase risk for heart disease and worsen outcomes in women.[34] In addition, men and women respond differently to different types of psychosocial stressors — for example, men who are married have lowered risk for heart disease but in women, marriage increases risk.[35]

Stress reduction is a key component to improving heart disease in women. In the SWITCHD trial, interventions to reduce stress in women were evaluated and researchers found that a group-based stress reduction program resulted in a lower risk of death in women with heart disease.[36] As compared to those women in the standard treatment group, those that participated in a psychosocial intervention designed to reduce stress were found to have a seven-year mortality rate of 7% (as compared to 30% in the standard therapy group). It is clear that stress reduction

---

[34] Dimsdale, J. E. (2008). Psychological stress and cardiovascular disease. *J Am Coll Cardiol*, Volume 51, 1237–1246.

[35] Nealey-Moore, J. B., Smith, T. W., Uchino, B. N. *et al.* (2007). Cardiovascular reactivity during positive and negative marital interactions. *J Behav Med*, Volume 30, 505–519.

[36] Orth-Gomér, K. (2009). Stress reduction prolongs life in women with coronary disease,The Stockholm Women's Intervention Trial for Coronary Heart Disease (SWITCHD). *Circulation: Cardiovascular Quality and Outcomes*, Volume 2, 25–32.

is an important part of prevention of heart disease. In women, the effects of different types of stressors may be different than those of men — we must continue to individualize treatment in order to maximize outcomes.

What are effective stress reduction techniques for women?

There are numerous publications and techniques for stress reduction available. The key is to determine what works best for each individual and what each person can incorporate into their daily routines. More common stress reduction tips include:

1. Meditate: Meditation can be a critical component for stress reduction. It allows you to be alone with your thoughts and focus on nothing but your own body. Meditation can be helpful in lowering heart rate and blood pressure and can be learned quickly. Some experts argue that daily five-minute meditation sessions can be quite successful.
2. Breathe deeply: Deep breathing or relaxation breathing can be used on its on or as a part of meditation. It can be incredibly effective in lowering both blood pressure and heart rate. Often, when we feel overwhelmed by stress, a moment of breathing exercises can significantly improve the way our bodies respond to stress.
3. Socialize/Social support: Having someone to talk to about life's stresses is another effective way to handle stress better. By verbalizing our feelings and sharing common experiences with others, patients are often better able to handle challenges and ultimately improve their coping mechanisms.
4. Exercise: Exercise is critical to cardiac health. Obviously, exercise helps reduce obesity and improves cardiovascular fitness. In addition, exercise can also help patients to manage stress better. Exercise is a great way to relax and spend time "alone with your thoughts".

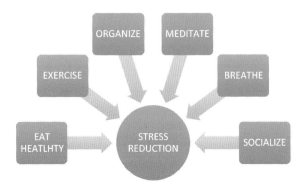

Figure 9.3   Strategies for stress reduction.

5. Organize and plan: Much of what contributes to stress is the fear of the unknown and uncertainty in the lives of our patients. By organizing and creating a family plan, many of the stressors can be relieved. Specifically, creating a family budget can help reduce the stress associated with financial pressures and obligations.

6. Eat healthily: Healthy eating can make an enormous difference in the way in which we all feel. Healthy nutritional choices can actually affect mood. Excessive junk food consumption has been associated with depression and anxiety.

Ultimately, we must empower women to take control of their own cardiovascular health through education and increasing awareness of risk. Obesity and stress can play an important role in the development and exacerbation of cardiovascular disease. By modifying diet and working to manage stress more effectively, women can make a significant difference in their own risk profiles for heart disease. As healthcare professionals we must provide support and counseling as our female patients set goals and develop plans for change.

Chapter Ten

Special Considerations: Women and Sudden Cardiac Death

As we have seen throughout this book, women are at significant risk for cardiovascular disease. Women are undertreated and under-served and often do not receive the same therapy as their male counterparts. Sudden cardiac death (SCD) is an unfortunate but frequent complication associated with coronary artery disease (CAD). It is estimated by the American Heart Association (AHA) in their 2014 report that nearly 425,000 people die suddenly from SCD in the US alone annually.[1] In fact, the AHA estimates that nearly 1,000 people suffer non-traumatic cardiac arrests outside of hospitals every single day — the survival rate is only around 5–10%. Only 60% of these arrests are treated by the emergency medical system (EMS) and, of these, nearly 25% were found to have a rhythm such as ventricular fibrillation (VF) or ventricular tachycardia (VT). Either of these rhythms would be easily treated with a shock from an implantable cardioverter-defibrillator (ICD) or an automatic external defibrillator (AED). When bystander CPR is

---

[1]AHA (2014). Statistical Update Heart Disease and Stroke Statistics — 2014 Update. A Report from the American Heart Association Circulation. Volume 129, e28–e292.

initiated survival rates significantly increase, and if an AED is present the rates may exceed 70%.

Sudden cardiac death in the US kills more people than all types of cancer combined. While women often worry about acquiring uterine or breast cancer, they are far more likely to die from cardiovascular disease. As we have seen earlier in this book, both women and their healthcare providers are often not aware of their greatest health threat — heart disease and its related complications. We have made great strides in developing important life-saving technologies that are useful in the treatment of heart disease and in the prevention of sudden cardiac death. However, it is frustrating to note that there is inequity in the way in which these therapies are applied to patients — there appears to be a significant gender bias.

ICDs have been used in humans since 1980 when the first human implant was performed.[2] A short time later in 1985, the FDA approved the device for routine implantation and expanded access of the device to patients all over the country. The device consists of a lead (or wire) that is placed inside the heart via a blood vessel, as well as an ICD generator which is implanted inside the chest. The generator is an advanced computer that monitors heart rate and rhythm and can react to abnormalities in heart rhythm with either pacing or a life-saving shock. Over the last 30 years, there have been numerous improvements in functionality and performance. ICDs have become widely accepted as life-saving therapy for patients with heart disease that have lowered ejection fractions (less than 35%) and are listed by the American College of Cardiology as class-I indications in many cases. When compared to other at-risk patients without ICD therapy, risk of death is lowered by nearly 30%.

It is clear that ICDs save lives — in both primary and secondary prevention of SCD. Evidence from numerous clinical trials including

---

[2] Mirowski, M., Reid, P. R., Mower, M. M. *et al.* (1980). Termination of malignant ventricular arrhythmias with an implanted automatic defibrillator in human beings. *N Engl J Med*, Volume 303, 322–324.

the Multicenter Automatic Defibrillator Implantation Trial (MADIT)-I, MADIT-II and the Sudden Cardiac Death in Heart Failure Trial (SCD-HeFT) make it quite clear — in patients who meet particular criteria and are at risk for SCD who are implanted with ICDs, survival is improved.[3-5] In patients who have survived an out-of-hospital cardiac arrest, data from the Antiarrhythmics versus Automatic Implantable Defibrillator Trial (AVID), suggests that ICD therapy should be considered first-line therapy in the secondary prevention of SCD.[6] In addition, ICDs have been proven to be effective and incredibly cost-effective — in secondary prevention the number of patients that need to be treated to save one life was determined to be 12 patients over two years. The average cost of treatment therefore becomes just 66,000 dollars for each life saved.[7]

The implantation of an ICD once included a thoracotomy where the leads were placed directly on the epicardial surface of the heart. Patients were often hospitalized for days after the procedure. Today, most devices can be implanted under conscious sedation utilizing a very small incision in the chest and the leads

---

[3]Moss, A. J., Hall, W. J., Cannom, D. S. *et al.* (1996). Multicenter Automatic Defibrillator Implantation Trial Investigators. Improved survival with an implanted defibrillator in patients with coronary disease at high risk for ventricular arrhythmia. *N Engl J Med*, Volume 335(26), 1933–1940.

[4]Moss, A. J., Zareba, W., Hall, W. J. *et al.* (2002). Prophylactic implantation of a defibrillator in patients with myocardial infarction and reduced ejection fraction. *N Engl J Med*, Volume 346(12), 877–883.

[5]Bardy, G. H., Lee, K. L., Mark, D. B. *et al.* (2005). Amiodarone or an implantable cardioverter-defibrillator for congestive heart failure. *N Engl J Med*, Volume 352(3), 225–237.

[6]Antiarrhythmics versus Implantable Defibrillators (AVID) Investigators (1997). A comparison of antiarrhythmic- drug therapy with implantable defibrillators in patients resuscitated from near-fatal ventricular arrhythmias. *N Engl J Med*, Volume 337(22), 1576–1583.

[7]Larsen, G., Hallstrom, A., McAnulty, J. *et al.* (2002). Cost-effectiveness of the implantable cardioverter-defibrillator versus antiarrhythmic drugs in survivors of serious ventricular tachyarrhythmias: Results of the Antiarrhythmics versus Implantable Defibrillators (AVID) economic analysis substudy. *Circulation*, Volume 105, 2049–2057.

are implanted in the heart via a percutaneous, trans-venous approach. In fact, most patients are able to go home after a one-night observation stay in the hospital. Over the last 20 years, indications for ICD implantation have expanded and hundreds of thousands of patients have benefited from device therapy. While the pool of ICD-eligible patients continues to increase, it has become clear that women are not implanted at the same rates as men with similar risk profiles. Data from numerous clinical trials show that women are under-represented in ICD registries and are much less likely to receive appropriate therapy.

In spite of an enormous body of evidence supporting the use of ICDs in the prevention of sudden cardiac death, women are not treated as aggressively as men. In a landmark trial published in *Journal of the American Medical Association* in 2007, a Medicare database was analyzed in order to determine if there were any gender-based differences in the utilization of ICD therapy for both primary and secondary prevention. In the study, it was found that women were much less likely to be referred for implantation of ICD devices even when they met the exact same criteria as men.[8] When men were compared with women who met criteria for primary prevention ICD implantation and secondary prevention ICD implantation, men were 3.2 and 2.4 times, respectively, more likely to receive a ICD therapy.

Why do women suffer from disparities in ICD utilization?

There are numerous theories as to why women are less likely to be implanted with an ICD even though they meet the same criteria as men. As we have discussed earlier in the book, women often present later with more significant and more widespread disease. Women often have more co-morbidities and are more likely to suffer in hospital complications. The prevalence of diabetes,

---

[8] Curtis, L. H., al-Khatid, S. M., Shea, A. M. *et al.* (2007). Sex differences in the use of implantable cardioverter-defibrillators for primary and secondary prevention of sudden cardiac death. *JAMA*, Volume 298(13), 1517–1524.

hypertension and peripheral vascular disease seems to be higher in women as compared to men undergoing the same procedures. In a paper by MacFadden *et al.* from the *Annals of Internal Medicine*, researchers attempted to identify factors that may influence ICD implantation in women.[9] After analysis of nearly 6,021 patients (half of whom were male), it was determined that women were more likely to suffer procedure-related complications as well as receive more inappropriate shocks from their device. In this registry, women were 1.7 times more likely to suffer complications at 45 days and nearly 31% less likely to receive appropriate ICD shock therapy.[9] As we have mentioned previously, women are more likely to suffer complications with other invasive cardiovascular procedures such as coronary artery bypass grafting and percutaneous revascularization procedures.[10] In order to balance risk with benefit, many physicians may be less likely to offer women invasive procedures in order to avoid complications. Peterson *et al.* found that women undergoing ICD implantation in the particular population of study were 31% more likely to suffer any adverse event as compared to men. More concerning is the fact that women were 71% more likely to suffer a major adverse event. Other studies have substantiated the higher complication rates with ICD implantation in women.[11] The reasons for the increased rate of complications, particularly with ICD, may very well have to do with anatomic considerations — smaller body size, smaller blood vessels and thinner right ventricular myocardium are likely to contribute to the higher rates of vascular damage and cardiac perforation seen in female patients undergoing implantation.

---

[9]MacFadden, D. R., Crystal, E., Krahn, A. D. *et al.* (2012). Sex Differences in implantable cardioverter-defibrillator outcomes: findings from a prospective defibrillator database. *Ann Intern Med*, Volume 156, 195–203.

[10]Jacobs, A. K. (2003). Coronary revascularization in women in 2003: sex revisited. *Circulation*, Volume 107, 375–377.

[11]Peterson, P. N., Daugherty, S. L., Wang, Y. *et al.* (2009). National cardiovascular data registry. Gender differences in procedure-related adverse events in patients receiving implantable cardioverter-defibrillator therapy. *Circulation*, Volume 119, 1078–1084.

What can physicians do to minimize risk?

Certainly, none of the data surrounding adverse events should be interpreted as a reason to *not* implant female patients with potentially life-saving devices. Rather, this data should motivate clinicians to improve care for women undergoing ICD implantation. Better technologies are in development with smaller lead and device sizes. It would stand to reason that smaller devices are likely to lead to fewer anatomic-related issues. Industry leaders in the development of devices must dedicate resources to making device therapy safer for both men and women. Moreover, implanting physicians must be aware of the greater risks for complications in women and be vigilant during the implant process. Healthcare providers who are considering referral of a female patient for implantation of an ICD must work to maximize success through effective treatments of co-morbidities in order to help optimize patients for the procedure.

The contribution of body image issues to ICD utilization in women

Certainly, the implantation of a medical device such as an ICD can have an impact on body image. For women, this impact may be greater than that experienced by men. Studies have shown that women who are considering ICD implantation may not be willing to proceed due to misconceptions about the appearance of the device in the chest and how others may perceive them. Data from the University of North Carolina indicates that women are more concerned with the appearance of the surgical scar and how it may affect the way clothes fit and their ability to wear a swimsuit.[12] In another study, Sowell *et al.* find that it is essential for healthcare providers to discuss alternative ICD implant techniques (such as

---

[12] Davis, L. L., Vitale, K. A., Irmiere, C. A. (2004). Body image changes associated with dual-chamber pacemaker insertion in women. *Heart and Lung, The Journal of Acute and Critical Care*, Volume 33(5), 273–280.

sub-pectoral implants, axillary implants, etc.) with female patients and allow them more time to make informed decisions concerning the procedure.[13] Alternative implantation techniques have been shown to be reliable and effective in long-term follow-up and provide the same risk reduction as standard implantation techniques and sites.[14] It is essential to provide both pre-operative and post-operative counseling and support for women undergoing ICD implantation in order to avoid any negative body image repercussions. In addition, providing information on the size and shape of the device and offering the possibility of plastic surgery input has been shown to be quite effective in helping women adapt well to ICD implantation.[15] As physicians and healthcare providers for women, it is essential that we are sensitive to the psychological issues surrounding the implantation of an ICD. Through engagement and sharing of information, we can ease patient worry and increase implantation rates for women.

More research is needed!

Ultimately, as healthcare providers, we must look for answers and derive ways to make ICD implantation safer for women. We know that ICDs save lives and that women are not referred for implantation at the same rate as men. It is essential that we carefully analyze the reasons behind increased complication rates and create new technology and interventions to improve safety. While many of the early trials in ICD therapy included a pre-dominance of male subjects, we must design trials composed of female

[13] Sowell, L. V., Kuhl, E. A., Sears, S. F. (2006). Device implant technique and consideration of body image: specific procedures for implantable cardioverter defibrillators in female patients. *J Womens Health*, Volume 15(7), 830–835.

[14] Obeyesekere, M. N., Kamberi, S., Youngs, N. *et al.* (2010). Long-term performance of submammary defibrillator system. *Europace*, Volume 12(9), 1239–1244.

[15] Walkerm, R. L., Campbell, K. A., Sears, S. F. *et al.* (2004). Women and the Implantable Cardioverter Defibrillator: A lifespan perspective on key psychosocial issues. *Clin Cardiol*, Volume 27, 543–546.

patients and explore gender-specific interventions to improve outcomes, reduce complications and improve care. In order to better treat female patients with arrhythmias we must reach a better understanding of the specific ways in which interventions such as ICDs impact women as compared to men. It is clear that biologic differences can make an enormous impact on the effectiveness and safety of particular therapies. As medicine moves into the next decade, personalized medicine and patient-specific therapies will be the norm — it is my hope that these types of interventions will foster the equal treatment of individuals, irrespective of gender, race or socioeconomic status.

Chapter Eleven

Women and Congestive Heart Failure

Congestive heart failure (CHF) is a severe consequence of cardio-vascular disease. In general CHF can be caused by coronary artery disease (CAD) and myocardial infarction (MI) as well as a plethora of other non-ischemic factors. CHF is the number one cause of hospitalization in the US today and accounts for billions of dollars in healthcare expenditures each year. In the setting of CAD and post-MI, the lifetime risk for the development of CHF is identical in men and women and is roughly one in five. However, in non-MI CHF, the lifetime risk is much higher in women than in men — one in six as compared to one in nine.[1] Most experts agree that other causes of CHF, such as long-standing, untreated hypertension, may be to blame for the high rate of non-MI-related CHF in women. Many women do not adequately address basic health issues such as treatment of hypertension and this may explain the disproportionately high rates of CHF in women. There have been multiple epidemiological studies that have suggested that there may be gender differences in progression and prognosis in CHF

---

[1] Lloyd-Jones, D. M. (2002). Lifetime risk for developing congestive heart failure: The Framingham Heart Study. *Circulation*, Volume 106, 3068–3072.

once it develops.[2] The reasons for these gender differences in prognosis are not clear — it may be that women present later with more severe left ventricular dysfunction and more advanced CHF.

Data has shown that women tend to present later with CHF and often have more diastolic dysfunction than men. In addition, female patients with CHF have greater functional impairment, more hospitalizations, overall lower quality of life and increased rates of depression when compared to men with similar disease burdens.[3, 4] Women are much more likely to have CHF with preserved left ventricular function but do seem to have overall lower mortality rates.

To put these statistics in perspective, a woman's lifetime risk of developing breast cancer is one in nine — much lower than the lifetime risk of CHF.[5] As mentioned previously in the book, women tend to believe that their greatest health risk comes from breast and uterine cancer when, in reality, their greatest risk is from heart disease and its complications. With improved treatments for heart disease and other medical advancements that are promoting longevity in the population, it is expected that the rates of CHF will continue to grow at an alarming rate. Strategies have been developed to work at primary prevention of CHF related to hypertension and seem to be effective — some studies even tout a 50% reduction in incidence of CHF in populations where hypertension is aggressively managed.[6] We now have well-proven therapies for

---

[2] Ho, K. K., Anderson, K. M., Kannel, W. B. *et al.* (1993). Survival after the onset of congestive heart failure in Framingham Heart Study subjects. *Circulation*, Volume 88, 107–115.

[3] Deswal, A. and Bozkurt, B. (2006). Comparison of morbidity in women versus men with heart failure and preserved ejection fraction. *Am J Cardiol*, Volume 97, 1228–1231.

[4] Gottlieb, S. S., Khatta, M., Friedmann, E. *et al.* (2004). The influence of age, gender, and race on the prevalence of depression in heart failure patients. *J Am Coll Cardiol*, Volume 43, 1542–1549.

[5] Feuer, E. J., Wung, L., Boring, C. C. *et al.* (1993). The lifetime risk of developing breast cancer. *J Natl Cancer Inst*, Volume 85, 892–897.

[6] Senni, M., Triboiuilloy, C. M., Rodeheffer, R. J. *et al.* (1999). Congestive heart failure in the community: Trends in incidence and survival in a 10-year period. *Arch Intern Med*, Volume 159, 29–34.

the treatment of acute MI. In addition, drugs such as ACE inhibitors and beta-blockers — when used properly in the post-MI period — will promote remodeling of the heart muscle and ultimately reduce the incidence of CHF.

Common causes of CHF

Congestive heart failure has many identified causes. CHF can either be due to systolic dysfunction or related to diastolic or relaxation abnormalities. Both varieties are associated with significant morbidity and mortality as well as extensive costs to the healthcare system. In systolic dysfunction, the left ventricular ejection fraction is reduced and the ventricle is no longer able to meet the demands of contraction and perfusion — resulting in congestion, edema and clinical symptoms consistent with CHF. In diastolic dysfunction, certain insults result in the impairment of ventricular relaxation during diastole and subsequent congestion and similar clinical symptoms. The more common etiologies of CHF are varied but include:

1. Coronary artery disease/Ischemic heart disease
2. Hypertension
3. Valvular heart disease
4. Idiopathic dilated cardiomyopathy
5. Congenital heart disease
6. Infiltrative disease (sarcoidosis, amyloidosis)
7. Others (anemia, thyroid disease, etc)

While the most common etiology appears to be CAD, each of these disorders can produce CHF to some degree — all are associated with significant morbidity and mortality.

Coronary artery disease: CAD and post-MI CHF is quite common. In the setting of CAD and MI, the patient's left ventricular ejection fraction is reduced due to infarction and necrosis of healthy cardiac myocytes during an acute cardiovascular event. During the post-MI period, much of the formerly healthy heart muscle is replaced with scar and fibrous tissue. These areas of infarction, if extensive, can impair the overall contractility of the heart. In some circumstances, such as when the area of the heart containing the left bundle branch is involved, the contractility of the heart can become dyssynchronous — further impairing the efficiency of the heart during systole.

Hypertension: Hypertension is one of the more common causes of CHF.[7] In the setting of long-standing hypertension, the heart makes adaptive changes over time. According to Starling's law of the heart, there comes a point at which the muscle cells can no longer continue to compensate for the increased wall stress and pressure that is imparted by elevated arterial pressures. The heart can become dilated and the ejection fraction can fall — systolic CHF then ensues. Alternatively, the heart can become stiff and relaxation is limited, resulting in diastolic heart failure. Prognosis following the onset of hypertension-related CHF is poor — according to a study in *JAMA*, only 24% of men and 31% of women were alive five years after diagnosis.[8]

Valvular heart disease: Valvular heart disease can have different effects on the heart and can result in clinical CHF. Depending on the particular type of valvular abnormality, symptoms can range from mild to severe CHF and can develop slowly over time or present acutely and in dramatic fashion. Most CHF associated with vavlular heart disease is systolic in nature, although there are situations that may produce relaxation abnormalities and result in diastolic CHF. The most common valvular lesions associated with the development of CHF are aortic stenosis and mitral regurgitation and tend to occur more frequently in patients over the age of 65.[9]

---

[7] Levy, D., Larson M. G., Vasan, R. S. *et al.* (1996). The progression from hypertension to congestive heart failure. *JAMA*, Volume 275, 1557–1562.

[8] *Ibid.*

[9] Rich, M. W. (1997). Epidemiology, pathophysiology, and etiology of congestive heart failure in older adults. *Journal of the American Geriatrics Society*, Volume 45(8), 968–974.

Interestingly, a study from *The Lancet* in 2006 indicates that even though prevalence of disease is similar and not gender specific, women are less likely to be diagnosed with and treated for valvular heart disease.[10]

Idiopathic dilated cardiomyopathy (IDCM): IDCM is common in the world today. In nearly 50% of cases of CHF, the etiology remains unknown and these patients are often termed idiopathic cardiomyopathies.[11] IDCM may be caused by numerous agents, including infection, toxic insults, genetic/inherited conditions, as well as inflammatory mediated events. In women, an important clinical syndrome associated with IDCM is the peri-partum cardiomyopthy (PPCM). In PPCM, women develop symptoms of CHF within the last month of pregnancy or within five months of delivery and left ventricular dysfunction is often severe. These pregnancy-related cardiomyopathies have a variable course — some resolve with delivery whereas others begin and persist in the post-partum period.[12] PPCM occurs in women with no pre-existing cardiovascular disease.

Congenital heart disease (CHD): As therapies for CHD continue to improve, many patients are living well into adulthood with significant congenital lesions. Over time, some of these patients do in fact develop left ventricular dysfunction and CHF related to their particular CHD lesion. In addition, women with CHD must be carefully managed during pregnancy as pregnancy-induced changes in the cardiovascular system can have particularly severe implications for women. In addition, women with CHD who are pregnant

---

[10]Nkomo, V. T. (2006). Burden of valvular heart diseases: A population-based study. *The Lancet*, Volume 368(9540), 1005–1011.

[11]Hazebroek, M. (2012). Idiopathic dilated cardiomyopathy: Possible triggers and treatment strategies. *Neth Heart J*, 20(7–8), 332–335.

[12]Pearson, G. D., Veille, J. C., Rahimtoola, S. *et al.* (2000). Peripartum cardiomyopathy: National Heart, Lung, and Blood Institute and Office of Rare Diseases (National Institutes of Health) workshop recommendations and review. *JAMA*, Volume 283, 1183–1188.

are at increased risk for offspring with CHD as compared to the general population.

Infiltrative diseases: Infiltrative diseases such as sarcoidosis and amyloidosis can produce restrictive cardiomyopathies. Patients with infiltrative diseases can have both diastolic as well as systolic dysfunction. These patients are at increased risk for ventricular arrhythmias and many present with syncope or sudden death syndromes at initial diagnosis.[13] Sarcoidosis occurs most commonly between the ages of 20 and 30 and is much more common in women than in men. Amyloidosis is a disease in which certain proteins are deposited in organs and replace normal healthy tissues with amyloid protein. In the case of cardiac amyloidosis, patients experience thickening of the left ventricle and often present with signs and symptoms consistent with CHF.

Other causes of CHF: Other diseases can contribute to the development of CHF. Some of these causes are quite reversible and may

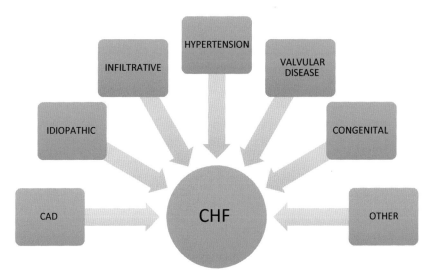

Figure 11.1   Common causes of CHF.

---

[13] Reuhl, J., Schneider, M., Sievert, H. *et al.* (1997). Myocardial sarcoidosis as a rare cause of sudden cardiac death. *Forensic Sci Int*, Volume 89(3), 145–153.

be related to metabolic abnormalities such as thyroid disease. Thyroid disease and related CHF is more common in women than in men. Other causes include severe anemia and viral infections (such as coxackievirus). Rare contributing factors include abnormalities of iron metabolism such as hemochromatosis, as well as inflammatory processes that result in a global myocarditis. While the above is not exhaustive, it does address most of the known causes of CHF.

Common symptoms associated with CHF

CHF can manifest in many different ways. Most commonly CHF symptoms are related to congestion and include shortness of breath, dyspnea on exertion and edema. Although the symptoms of CHF are similar in men and women, females tend to have more shortness of breath and peripheral edema as compared to their male counterparts. In addition, women also have more difficulty with exertional dyspnea as compared to men.

The cardinal signs and symptoms of CHF include:

1. Shortness of breath
2. Fatigue
3. Dyspnea on exertion
4. Peripheral edema
5. Positional nocturnal dyspnea and orthopnea
6. Cough

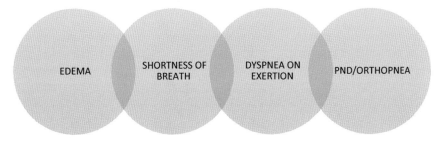

Figure 11.2 Common symptoms of CHF. PND = postural nocturnal dyspnea.

Symptoms may be slowly progressive or may occur very quickly, depending on the etiology of CHF.

Gender differences in risk factor effects

Not all risk factors have equivalent effects in both men and women. As clinicians and as patients, we must consider risk factors in the context of their variable gender-specific effects on lifetime risk for CHF. It is important to understand the impact of different risk factors on women and prioritize interventions in order to make the biggest impact on risk reduction in female patients.

Common risk factors for CHF include CAD, hypertension, diabetes, obesity, elevated cholesterol and smoking.[14] These risk factors

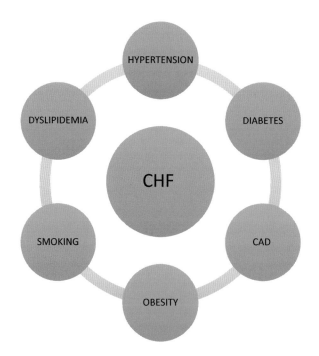

Figure 11.3   Risk factors for CHF.

[14] Petrie, M. C. (1999). Failure of women's hearts. *Circulation*, Volume 99, 2334–2341.

seem to have important gender-specific effects. For example, hypertension confers much greater risk for CHF in women than in men. Although the exact mechanism by which hypertension affects women differently is not known, it may be that the afterload increase that occurs with hypertension has a greater effect on women's hearts and results in more ventricular dysfunction — predisposing females to more CHF.[15] Interestingly, CAD is more prevalent in men with CHF as compared to women. Myocardial infarction is a much more common risk factor for CHF in men — however, in women who do have CAD and suffer a MI, CHF is much more common.[16] In addition, women who have had an MI and subsequently have been revascularized with coronary artery bypass grafting (CABG) are much more likely to develop CHF than men.[17] The presence of diabetes appears to have a very powerful effect for the development of CHF in women. Numerous studies have shown a direct correlation between the presence of diabetes and the development of CHF. When the rates of concomitant diabetes in women with CHF are compared to similar male patients, women had an eight-fold increase in incident heart failure and men only a four-fold increase. Although no mechanism for this effect is known, based on Framingham data, it is postulated that diabetes may produce increased wall thickness and left ventricular mass specific to women — thus contributing to diastolic relaxation abnormalities and clinical CHF in women.[18] In general, smoking appears to have a greater effect on men than in women — in fact, smoking appears to be less common in female CHF patients

---

[15] Garavaglia, G. E., Messerli, F. H., Schmieder, R. E. *et al.* (1989). Sex differences in cardiac adaptation to essential hypertension. *Eur Heart J*, Volume 10, 1110–1114.

[16] Tofler, G. H., Stone, P. H., Mueller, J. E. *et al.* (1987). Effects of gender and race on prognosis after myocardial infarction: Adverse prognosis for women, particularly black women. *J Am Coll Cardiol*, Volume 9, 473–482.

[17] Hoffman, R. M., Psaty, B. M. and Kronmal, R.A. (1994). Modifiable risk factors for incident heart failure in the Coronary Artery Surgery Study. *Arch Intern Med*, Volume 154, 417–423.

[18] Galderisi, M., Andersson, K. M., Wilson, P. W. F. *et al.* (1991). Echocardiographic evidence for the existence of a distinct diabetic cardiomyopathy: The Framingham Heart Study. *Am J Cardiol*, Volume 68, 85–89.

than in men — although some studies have shown that smoking seems to increase CHF risk in young men and older women with CHF.[19, 20] Obesity has been found to confer increased risk for CHF in both sexes, however, data from Framingham suggests that women who are obese may suffer even greater risk.[10,11] Dyslipidemia has also been associated with a higher risk for CHF in women as compared to men.

Sex differences in response to therapy for CHF

Historically, most CHF trials have included a minority of women as subjects. Much of the data that we use today to recommend therapy are not gender specific due to under-representation of women in the clinical trials. However, the best available data suggests that we should treat men and women in a similar fashion (until such time as gender-specific trials in CHF are conducted and published). Several clinical investigations have noted a difference in the way in which men and women respond to particular therapies. For example, men tend to gain a larger survival benefit from ACE inhibitors as compared to women.[21] In addition, meta-analysis of ACE inhibitor trials does indicate that women with CHF who are symptomatic derive more benefit from ACE inhibitors than those who were asymptomatic.[22] Certain angiotensin receptor blockers (ARBs) such as candesartan and valsartan appear to be beneficial in women and have been shown to reduce cardiovascular death and hospitalization

---

[19] Kannel, W. B. (1989). Epidemiological aspects of heart failure. *Cardiol Clin*, Volume 7, 1–9.

[20] Kannel, W. B. and Belanger, A. J. (1991). Epidemiology of heart failure. *Am Heart J*, Volume 121, 951–957.

[21] Petrie, M. C., Dawson, N. F., Murdoch, D. R. *et al.* (1999). Failure of women's hearts. *Circulation*, Volume 99, 2334–2341.

[22] Shekelle, P. G., Rich, M. W., Morton, S. C. *et al.* (2003). Efficacy of angiotensin-converting enzyme inhibitors and beta-blockers in the management of left ventricular systolic dysfunction according to race, gender, and diabetic status: a meta-analysis of major clinical trials. *J Am Coll Cardiol*, Volume 41, 1529–1538.

in women.[23] Some studies indicate that women have greater responses from beta-blockers due to sex-related differences in the way in which the drugs act *in vivo* — differences in pharmacokinetics may result in greater drug exposure in women.[24] The combination of beta-blockers and ACE inhibitors seems to be particularly effective in female patients with CHF. In this case, even though women and men may take the same dose of beta-blockers, women seem to achieve a greater benefit and ultimately may have better responses to beta-blockers in CHF.

Special circumstances: depression and CHF

Depression has been associated with CHF and the effective treatment of depression in CHF patients has had a significant impact on hospitalization and outcomes. The overall prevalence of depression in CHF ranges from 24% to 42%.[25] Numerous studies have also shown that the prevalence in depression among patients hospitalized with CHF is significantly higher in women.[26] More concerning is the fact that CHF patients with major depression are than twice as likely to die or be readmitted to the hospital as compared to those without depression at all.[27] Clearly, depression represents a major determinant of outcome in CHF — however,

[23]Young, J. B., Dunlap, M. E., Pfeffer, M. A. *et al.* (2004). Mortality and morbidity reduction with Candesartan in patients with chronic heart failure and left ventricular systolic dysfunction: Results of the CHARM low-left ventricular ejection fraction trials. *Circulation*, Volume 110, 2618–2626.

[24]Luzier, A. B., Killian, A., Wilton, J. H. *et al.* (1999). Gender-related effects on meto- prolol pharmacokinetics and pharmacodynamics in healthy volunteers. *Clin Pharmacol Ther*, Volume 66, 594–601.

[25]Havranek, E. P., Ware, M. G. and Lowes, B. D. (1999). Prevalence of depression in congestive heart failure. *Am J Cardiol*, Volume 84, 348–350.

[26]Freedland, K. E. (2003). Prevalence of depression in hospitalized patients with congestive heart failure. *Psychosomatic Medicine*, Volume 65(1), 119–128.

[27]Jiang, W., Alexander, J., Christopher, E. *et al.* (2001). Relationship of depression to increased risk of mortality and rehospitalization in patients with congestive heart failure. *Arch Intern Med*, Volume 161(15), 1849–1856.

many patients are not diagnosed or adequately treated. As health-care providers who treat patients with CHF, we must become more vigilant and work to ensure that we identify patients at risk for depression and provide them with proper therapies for depression once it is identified.

Chapter Twelve

Empowering Women to Take Control

Heart disease in women claims more lives than all types of cancer combined. Each year more than 600,000 patients die of heart disease in the US, and many of these victims are female. While death rates in men are declining, mortality in women continues to rise or stay the nearly the same. A large number of female patients never even knew that they were at risk for cardiovascular disease. Few had ever been screened for heart disease and most were undiagnosed and untreated. Like many women, these victims thought that they were more likely to die of breast cancer than of heart disease. Many incorrectly believed that heart disease was a disease of men.

Unfortunately, the legacy of limited awareness of heart disease in women persists in the US and the UK today. Although great strides have been made over the last decade, women with heart disease remain undertreated and underserved. As we have seen in previous chapters, there are many reasons for the gender-related disparities in care — some biologic, some societal and others related to healthcare provider attitudes and preconceived notions. Fortunately, I believe that there are several potential solutions that will allow us to close this unacceptable gap in care going forward. Working with patients, specialists and primary care providers in a more cooperative fashion will allow for earlier identification, screening and treatment of women who are at risk. However, in order to be successful in achieving our goals of equality in cardiovascular care, we must also engage patients and their families. Through education and awareness campaigns and activities, we must empower women to take control of their own cardiovascular health. Empowering patients to assume individual responsibility for their own heart health most often results in improved outcomes. Patients who are empowered are more likely to educate others and advocate for improved care for both themselves and their friends and families.

In order to understand better how we can empower women to take reduce their own risk for cardiovascular disease and its negative health consequences, we must first understand better what empowerment is all about. The concept of empowerment can be quite complex. In general, empowerment can be defined as a multi-dimensional process that allows people to take better control over their lives. Empowerment involves addressing interrelated social, economic and psychological issues and must occur at multiple levels — individual, group and community. The process of empowerment is a *journey* and allows individuals to implement change in their own lives, the lives of others and in society as a whole. In order to be relevant and effect change, empowerment must resolve around an issue that a person deems to be of significant importance. Patient empowerment has become a top priority in many countries including the US and the UK. When healthcare professionals involve the patient in care and treatment decisions, the physicians become more responsive to patients' needs and concerns and ultimately deliver better care. Moreover, patient compliance rates are increased when they are more closely involved in their own care plan.

What are some empowerment strategies for women?

Patient empowerment is a process designed to facilitate self-directed behavioral and lifestyle changes. Empowerment involves several steps. Much of the literature on empowerment of patients comes from diabetes education. For years, endocrinologists and diabetes educators have realized that blood sugar control and compliance is much improved through patient empowerment.[1] In the literature, empowerment involves providing the self-awareness and knowledge required for patients to understand their disease or risk for disease and ultimately provide self-care in consultation with a medical professional. This type of empowerment engages patients to participate in their own disease management. In the case of diabetes, patients are first educated about their disease and on its day-to-day management. They are taught what to look out for and what types of signs and symptoms may signify a medical emergency. They are then educated on how to best care for their diabetes and how to respond to changes in blood sugar levels or other potential complications. Once the patient is fully educated, they begin the process of understanding the principles of self-care and learn how to manage their day-to-day activities in the setting of chronic disease (in this case, diabetes). Once comfortable with the routine management, patients begin to take control of their own diabetes care and learn to interact with their healthcare professional when necessary — in a team-based approach to care. Patient engagement and involvement in daily care between visits with healthcare providers has been shown to substantially improve blood sugar control and decrease diabetic-related complications. Similarly, women with heart disease or risk factors for disease can be empowered through the same process in a stepwise fashion — awareness, education, engagement and ultimately patient empowerment to effect *change*.

In the case of women with heart disease (or at risk for heart disease) the process of empowerment involves improving community awareness of the risks of heart disease to women. Women must

---

[1]Anderson, R. M., Funnell, M. M., Barr, P. A. *et al.* (1991). Learning to empower patients: results of professional education program for diabetes educators. *Diabetes Care*, Volume 14(7), 584–590.

be educated that they are at risk for disease and that they are more likely to die from heart disease than any other medical problem. In addition, women who do not have heart disease must be made aware of the risk factors for heart disease and how each individual woman can modify her risk. As mentioned in previous chapters, these important educational objectives can be handled through multiple venues — community seminars, internet sites and social media, as well as direct person-to-person contact. Once women have been informed of the facts surrounding heart disease and the risk factors associated with developing disease, they must be provided with goals and instructions as to how to modify risk. Once they have understood the problem, its risks and how to modify risk they become empowered to effect change. Through mass education and community-wide efforts, not only are those at risk empowered, but those who are not yet at risk are also educated and ready to assist others to modify lifestyle and limit risk for heart disease. As a society we must develop a culture of heart healthy living — the empowerment of women is critical to success in reducing death from heart disease in both the US and the UK. Ideally, we, as a society, create a "buzz" around our efforts to close the gender gap in care.

What steps can patients take to empower themselves?

Once we have empowered women to make changes in lifestyle and (hopefully) encourage others around them (including friends and family) to do the same, we must continue to engage patients in their own care. Women must begin to take control of their own healthcare. For instance, if a woman is seeing a provider that she does not connect with and does not feel partnered with, she must make a change. Traditionally, it is very difficult for patients (male or female) to "fire" their physician. However, it is critical that each individual female have a partner in care that they can work effectively with. Success in prevention of disease is dependent upon a close relationship with a healthcare provider in order to achieve common goals. Each patient must have find a physician or other healthcare provider with whom they are able to feel comfortable asking questions, debating treatments and "co-managing" disease. It is no longer acceptable for a patient to sit back and let the physician make all of the decisions for her — each patient must play an active and engaged role in care. Each patient must not only accept individual responsibility for her own care and disease management but must also advocate for herself and her family.

Physicians and other providers of healthcare to women must be open to discussion: we must be willing to listen more and dictate care less. It is vital that we take the time to understand the patient and their family. It is critical that we also understand what things are important to the patients and what they value most. Through a better understanding of each individual's circumstances we may be better equipped to help guide them through their healthcare journey. Ultimately, physicians must move away from algorithmic approaches to care. We must certainly apply the guidelines and best practices to each case *but* we must bond with each patient and treat each individual in a way that best suits their particular risks, goals and needs.

Here are a few important tips to enhance productivity and success for patients and healthcare providers when preparing for an office visit:

1. *Come prepared*: Patients should have read about their disease and come with questions. Providers must be ready to answer and take the time required to make sure that they are meeting the needs of the patient and addressing the concerns, fears and uncertainties that each patient may bring to the visit.

2. *Be accountable*: Both physician and patient should have "action items" assigned at the office visit and be held accountable for reporting the results to one another at subsequent visits. For example — the physician may be responsible for checking a cholesterol level and reporting the findings and the patient may be responsible for attending an exercise program three times a week during the interval between visits. This type of

shared responsibility can motivate and empower patients to improve their own cardiac health. They are engaged, informed and active participants.

3. *Be ready to negotiate*: Patients and physicians are not always going to agree. We must work to provide our female patients with an atmosphere in the clinic that promotes shared responsibility and negotiation. There are often multiple ways to approach a particular problem — it is important to choose the treatment that is acceptable to both doctor and patient — success rates will be improved.

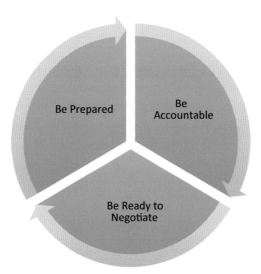

Figure 12.1   Keys to successful navigation of a visit with a healthcare provider.

How will empowerment ultimately improve outcomes for women with heart disease?

I believe that empowerment of women is the most critical step in improving outcomes for women with heart disease. The empowerment of women will change the way in which physicians and other healthcare providers deliver care. Women with heart disease can set a healthy example for others who are yet to be diagnosed through effective secondary preventative efforts. Now, more than ever, women throughout the US and the UK are leaders in business, politics and education — by engaging these leaders in health promotion and individualizing healthcare for women we can change the course of heart disease and reduce cardiac-related morbidity and mortality over the next decade.

While we have certainly made improvements in cardiac care for women over the last decade, gender differences in care still remain. Through education, awareness and partnerships with engaged and empowered patients we can move closer towards equality in care and ultimately close the gap for the years to come.

Chapter Thirteen

Women and Atrial Fibrillation

Atrial fibrillation (AF) is the most common heart rhythm disorder in the world and is associated with stroke and peripheral embolism.[1] Nearly 2.5 million people in the US alone have AF and those with AF are five times more likely to suffer a stroke as compared to those without AF. As we age, the incidence of AF increases and risk factors for AF include advancing age, diabetes, hypertension CHF, valvular heart disease and myocardial infarction.[2] It has been long proven that AF is an independent risk factor for stroke and confers a three-to-five-fold increased risk that increases with age.[3] Data from the Framingham Heart Study demonstrates a nearly two-fold increase in death in patients with AF as compared to those without AF and this risk was present in both men and women.[4] Other trials such as the RACE study (RAte

---

[1]Wolf, P. A., Abbott, R. D. and Kannel W. B. (1991). Atrial fibrillation as an independent risk factor for stroke: the Framingham study. *Stroke*, Volume 22, 983–988.

[2]Benjamin, E. J., Levy, D., Vaziri, S. M. *et al.* (1994). Independent risk factors for atrial fibrillation in a population-based cohort: the Framingham Heart Study. *JAMA*. Volume 271, 840–844.

[3]Wolf, P. A., Abbott, R. D. and Kannel, W. B. (1991). Atrial fibrillation as an independent risk factor for stroke: the Framingham Study. *Stroke*, Volume 22, 983–988.

[4]Benjamin, E. J. (1998). Impact of atrial fibrillation on the risk of death: The Framingham Heart Study. *Circulation*, Volume 98, 946–952.

Control versus Electrical cardioversion) have demonstrated a higher mortality and lower quality of life in women with AF as compared to men.[5]

Pathophysiology, causes and symptoms of AF

AF occurs when the atria no longer participate in a coordinated electrical systole resulting in contraction. In AF, the cells in the atria rapidly depolarize and fire in a disordered fashion, resulting in the absence of P-waves on electrocardiography (EKG) and a variable R-R interval with fibrillatory oscillations on a rhythm strip. Symptoms of AF may be quite variable and may involve no symptoms whatsoever in some patients. In other individuals, there may be significant fatigue, shortness of breath, exercise intolerance or palpitations.

AF is associated with a number of toxic, metabolic, endocrine and genetic abnormalities and the incidence increases with age.[6] Thyroid disease is commonly identified as a precipitating factor. Some of the more common cardiac-related causes of AF include coronary artery disease, cardiothoracic surgery, hypertension and valvular heart disease. In addition, congenital heart disease can predispose patients to the development of AF at earlier ages. The etiologies of AF seem to differ in population studies of men and women. Men are more likely to have coronary artery disease and women are more likely to have hypertension and valvular heart disease as a predisposing factor for AF.

The causes of AF are multi-factorial and can be both primary and secondary to other medical problems.

---

[5] Rienstra, M., van Veldhuisen D. J., Hagens, V. E. *et al.* (2005). Gender-related differences in rhythm control treatment in persistent atrial fibrillation. *J Am Coll Cardiol*, Volume 46, 1298–1306.

[6] Kannel, W. B., Wolf, P. A., Benjamin, E. J. *et al.* (1998). Prevalence, incidence, prognosis, and predisposing conditions for atrial fibrillation: population-based estimates. *Am J Cardiol*, Volume 82, 2N–9N.

Treatment of AF

In AF, the goal of therapy is the prevention of stroke and the relief of symptoms. In many patients, most of the symptoms are related to poorly controlled, irregular ventricular rates.[7] Interestingly, the rates of death in patients with a history of AF is doubled — although this finding appears to be an association rather than a case of cause and effect. The treatment strategies for AF include either control of rate versus control of rhythm. However, a key component to either strategy is stroke prevention through anticoagulation. Data from the AFFIRM trial makes it abundantly clear that it is safe and effective to treat AF with either a rate control or rhythm control strategy with similar outcomes.[8] In patients in which a strategy of rhythm control is chosen, therapy most often includes initiation of antiarrhythmic drugs followed by electrical cardioversion.[9] Many clinicians argue that the rhythm control strategy offers the advantages of fewer symptoms, reduced risk of stroke (because of a presumed less time spent in AF), and eventual discontinuation of anticoagulation therapy. A potential disadvantage to a rhythm control strategy is the fact that antiarrhythmic therapy includes a higher risk of side effects (all antiarrhythmic drugs have the potential for pro-arrhythmia).[10] Alternatively, a strategy of rate control focuses on the use of drug therapy with AV (atrio-ventricular) nodal blocking agents to control ventricular response during AF. With this strategy, less toxic drugs may be utilized but chronic anticoagulation is a must. In addition, in

---

[7]Krahn, A. D., Manfreda, J., Tate, R. B. *et al.* (1995). The natural history of atrial fibrillation: incidence, risk factors, and prognosis in the Manitoba Follow-Up Study. *Am J Med*, Volume 98, 476–484.

[8]AFFIRM Investigators (2002). A comparison of rate control and rhythm control in patients with atrial fibrillation. *N Engl J Med*, Volume 347, 1825–1833.

[9]Falk, R. H. (2001). Atrial fibrillation. *N Engl J Med*, Volume 344, 1067–1078.

[10]Crijns, H. J., van Gelder, I. C., van Gilst, W. H. *et al.* (1991). Serial antiarrhythmic drug treatment to maintain sinus rhythm after electrical cardioversion for chronic atrial fibrillation or atrial flutter. *Am J Cardiol*, Volume 68, 335–341.

refractory cases of rate control in AF, an ablation of the AV node along with pacemaker implantation may be utilized in order to definitively control ventricular rates.

Over the last 15 years, newer, more advanced therapies for AF have been developed that can be utilized in conjunction with both the rate control and rhythm control strategies. Radiofrequency ablation is an invasive technique that focuses on eliminating the electrical triggers for AF in the left atrium and pulmonary veins.[11] In this procedure, catheters are taken to the left atrium via a percutaneus approach with a trans-septal puncture of the intra-atrial septum. The pulmonary veins are then carefully mapped and electrical triggers are eliminated through the application of radiofrequency energy. In many patients the cure rates for AF with this technique can approach 85% or more. Other invasive techniques have been utilized for rate control. In patients with chronic, refractory AF, many cardiologists will implant a pacemaker (or biventricular pacemaker) and subsequently ablate the AV node. In this procedure, the ablation of the AV node will eliminate all rapid ventricular response and will make the patient pacemaker-dependent. Because of the data surrounding right-ventricular-only pacing and increased incidence of congestive heart failure (CHF), many clinicians will implant a biventricular device in order to maintain ventricular synchrony and pace both the left and right ventricles — thus avoiding pacing-related CHF.[12,13] This technique can be incredibly effective and can produce patient responses and outcomes similar to those with rhythm control. However, in patients

---

[11] Haïssaguerre, M. (2002). Electrophysiological end point for catheter ablation of atrial fibrillation initiated from multiple pulmonary venous foci. *Circulation*, Volume 101, 1409–1417.

[12] DAVID Trial Investigators (2002). Dual-chamber pacing or ventricular backup pacing in patients with an implantable defibrillator the dual chamber and VVI implantable defibrillator. *JAMA*, Volume 288(24), 3115–3123.

[13] Doshi, R. N. (2005). Left ventricular-based cardiac stimulation post AV nodal ablation evaluation (the PAVE study). *J Cardiovasc Electrophysiol*, Volume 16(11), 1160–1165.

with chronic AF and AV node ablation, it is essential that lifelong anticoagulation is maintained in order to prevent stroke. In those who have successfully undergone AF ablation, it is possible to discontinue anticoagulation after a long period of proven maintenance of normal sinus rhythm (NSR).

Interestingly, as with coronary artery disease, there does appear to be stark differences in the treatment of men versus women. Data from the Euro Heart Survey on Atrial Fibrillation was analyzed and researchers found that women with AF were much less likely to be adequately anticoagulated (even though women seem to have a higher risk of AF-related stroke) and tended to be treated with a more conservative rate-control-only strategy.[14] In addition, women in this database were much less likely to undergo transesophogeal echocardiography to exclude a left atrial thrombus prior to electrical cardioversion and were also less likely to undergo stress testing as compared to men with similar clinical characteristics. Just as we have seen with the treatment of coronary artery disease, women with AF were also much less likely to undergo invasive procedures for AF such as catheter ablation.

AF and stroke

Stroke is the most common reason for the increased morbidity and mortality associated with AF and women at risk for stroke are often overlooked. In AF, the non-effective mechanical systole associated with the arrhythmia predisposes patients to form clots in the left atrial appendage. In many cases these thrombi will dislodge and produce stroke by occluding a cerebral artery. There is a great deal of data to suggest that anticoagulation can reduce the risk of stroke to that of patients without AF. Yet, many women with AF are not treated with proper anticoagulation.

---

[14] Dagres, N. (2007). Gender-related differences in presentation, treatment, and outcome of patients with atrial fibrillation in Europe. A report from the Euro Heart Survey on Atrial Fibrillation. *J Am Coll Cardiol*, Volume 49, 572–577.

Anticoagulation has been shown to be highly efficacious in the prevention of stroke — meta-analysis of several different trials demonstrated a 61% reduction in the incidence of stroke in patients treated with warfarin.[15] While bleeding complications are a real concern, the target anticoagulation level must balance risk of bleeding with stroke prevention. Bleeding complications increase with advanced age but anticoagulation is still indicated. There are several types of anticoagulation available including aspirin, warfarin and the newer direct thrombin inhibitors. Aspirin provides only modest stroke risk reduction as compared to the other agents but does appear to be more effective in patients with hypertension or diabetes.[16] Several trials over the last 20 years have shown that warfarin is clearly superior to aspirin in the prevention of stroke in AF and warfarin anticoagulation has become the standard of care for the prevention of thrombo-embolism.[17] Warfarin therapy requires frequent blood testing to monitor levels and effective blood levels can be affected by changes in diet and the use of certain concomitant drugs. Newer anticoagulants have been developed and FDA approved in the last several years that provide alternatives to warfarin therapy and have been shown to be either equivalent to warfarin or superior in terms of efficacy and safety.[18-20] The advantages of the newer

---

[15]Hart, R. G., Benavente, O., McBride, R. *et al.* (1991). Antithrombotic therapy to prevent stroke in patients with atrial fibrillation: a meta-analysis. *Ann Intern Med*, Volume 131, 492–501.

[16]The Atrial Fibrillation Investigators (1997). The efficacy of aspirin in patients with atrial fibrillation. Analysis of pooled data from 3 randomized trials. *Arch Intern Med*, Volume 157, 1237–1240.

[17]Anon (1991). Stroke prevention in atrial fibrillation study. Final results. *Circulation*, Volume 84, 527–539.

[18]Patel, M. R. and Mahaffey, K. W. (2011). Rivaroxaban versus warfarin in nonvalvular atrial fibrillation. *N Engl J Med*, Volume 365, 883–891.

[19]Granger, C. B. (2011). Apixaban versus warfarin in patients with atrial fibrillation. *N Engl J Med*, Volume 365, 981–992.

[20]Connolly, S. J. (2009). Dabigatran versus warfarin in patients with atrial fibrillation. *N Engl J Med*, Volume 361, 1139–1151.

anticoagulation agents are the fact that they do not require blood testing to monitor levels and they are not affected by diet. Drawbacks include the fact that there are no available reversal agents for these drugs.

Most clinicians utilize the CHADS2 score to determine the need for anticoagulation.[21] The CHADS2 score considers CHF, hypertension, age, diabetes and prior stroke in order to determine thromboembolic risk. With the CHADS2 score, a clinician is able to quickly calculate the lifetime risk for stroke in a patient with AF based on certain risk factors. By calculating this score, the healthcare provider is able to determine which anticoagulant regimen is best indicated for the individual patient.

Women and AF: future directions to improve outcome

Just as with the treatment of coronary artery disease, women with AF are often undertreated and underserved and therapy often falls below standard of care. Data from the *European Heart Journal* has indicated that as a group, women with AF are more likely to not be anticoagulated and seem to have higher rates of bleeding complication and debilitating stroke.[22] In addition, women with AF are not treated as aggressively and represent a minority of patients undergoing advanced procedures such as AF ablation and other device-based therapy. As healthcare providers, we must work diligently to ensure that women with AF are treated according to well-published guidelines. While it is true that women are more likely to suffer procedural-related complications, this should not preclude therapy for those who are

---

[21] Gage, B. F. (2001). Validation of clinical classification schemes for predicting stroke results from the national registry of atrial fibrillation. *JAMA*, Volume 285(22), 2864–2870.

[22] Gomberg-Maitland, M. (2006). Anticoagulation in women with nonvalvular atrial fibrillation in the stroke prevention using an oral thrombin inhibitor (SPORTIF) trials. *European Heart Journal*, Volume 27, 1947–1953.

indicated. Even though women with AF are more likely to suffer complications and excess morbidity, we must strive to individualize therapy and provide the best available treatments. Just as with coronary artery disease, we must work diligently to educate women about their risk for AF and how to prevent devastating consequences such as stroke. Educating the public as to the etiologies, symptoms and risks associated with atrial fibrillation must play a bigger role in public health policy. Particularly in the era of healthcare reform and cost containment, working to prevent disease must be of paramount importance.

Index

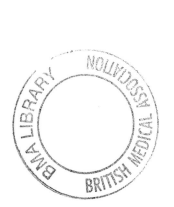